Current Approach to Acute and Emergency Infections

*Edited by Ozgur Karcioglu,
Canan Akman and Göksu Afacan Ozturk*

Published in London, United Kingdom

Current Approach to Acute and Emergency Infections
http://dx.doi.org/10.5772/intechopen.1006781
Edited by Ozgur Karcioglu, Canan Akman and Göksu Afacan Ozturk

Contributors
Albert Shakirov, Bilgen Ozkaya, Canan Akman, Chang-Wen Chen, Dragan Piljić, Ekaterina Soloveitchik, Farah Dedović, Feride Sinem Akgun, Göksu Afacan Ozturk, Hana Muslić, Haris Vranić, Haris Vukas, Ildar Lutfarakhmanov, Melica Imamović-Bošnjak, Omer Halit Keskin, Ozgur Karcıoglu, Peter Mironov, Ruvejda Dizdarević, Samra Kadić-Vukas, Sumeja Ćatić, Taner Karlidag

First published in London, United Kingdom, 2025 by IntechOpen
IntechOpen is the global imprint of INTECHOPEN LIMITED, registered in England and Wales, registration number: 11086078, 167-169 Great Portland Street, London, W1W 5PF, United Kingdom

For EU product safety concerns: IN TECH d.o.o., Prolaz Marije Krucifikse Kozulić 3, 51000 Rijeka, Croatia, info@intechopen.com or visit our website at intechopen.com.

British Library Cataloguing-in-Publication Data
A catalogue record for this book is available from the British Library

Current Approach to Acute and Emergency Infections
Edited by Ozgur Karcioglu, Canan Akman and Göksu Afacan Ozturk
p. cm.
Print ISBN 978-1-83634-743-9
Online ISBN 978-1-83634-742-2
eBook (PDF) ISBN 978-1-83634-744-6

Meet the editor

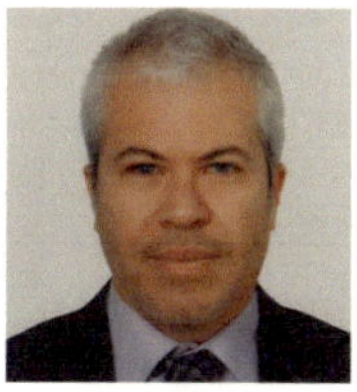

In 1994, Dr. Ozgur Karcioglu started residency at Dokuz Eylul University (DEU) Medical School, Department of Emergency Medicine. He completed the Fellowship Program in International EM at Pennsylvania State University (2005). He has served as the chairman of the department in DEU (2005-2007). He has been in charge of the ED of Bakirkoy Research and Training Hospital (2007-2009), and then a faculty member at Acıbadem University (2009-15). He is currently a full professor and chair at Taksim Education and Research Hospital in İstanbul. He has served as a founder and a board member of The Emergency Medical Association of Turkey (2007-2009). Around 200 articles of his were published in international journals. He has contributed to seven books as editor and authored 40 chapters. He serves as a member of the Editorial Board for several journals. He is also an instructor for the American Heart Association's Basic and Advanced Cardiac Life Support Courses.

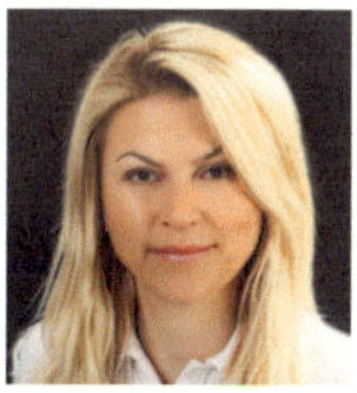

Canan Akman completed her specialization at Hacettepe University Faculty of Medicine, Department of Emergency Medicine, from 2006 to 2011. Between 2012 and 2016, she worked as an emergency medicine specialist and administrative manager of Kanuni Sultan Süleyman Training and Research Hospital. She is an active member of the toxicology, trauma, pediatric emergency, and geriatric working groups in the Emergency Medicine Association of Turkey (EMAT). She has been working as an education coordinator, Erasmus coordinator, and faculty board member at Çanakkale Onsekiz Mart University (ÇOMU) since 2021 and was appointed as an associate professor at the same institution in 2021. She is still serving as assistant chief physician in the hospital. At the same time, she completed her master's degree in Medical Education at the ÇOMU Institute of Educational Sciences in 2021. So far, she has published 51 articles and written 9 book chapters.

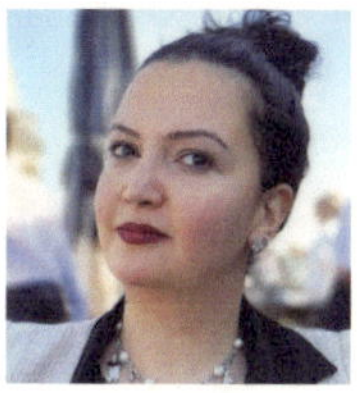

After completing her medical education at Marmara University in 2010, Göksu Afacan Ozturk received her Emergency Medicine Residency training at the Çanakkale Onsekiz Mart University (ÇOMU). She worked at Başkent University, Biruni University, and Istanbul Aydın University, respectively. She is currently working as an assistant professor at Istanbul Aydın University and Acıbadem Health Group. Apart from her articles published in three international and four national journals, she has published a total of eight book chapters. She is a member of the European Society for Emergency Medicine (EUSEM), as well as several Turkish associations. In addition to her certificates in various fields, she gave training courses in multiple cities in Turkey and abroad (Egypt, 2018) on Advanced Cardiac Life Support and the use of ultrasound in the ED.

Contents

Preface

In recent decades, the number of emergency visits with sepsis and severe infections has increased significantly. The most familiar sources of infection are the respiratory and urinary tracts, abdomen, skin, and soft tissue. Each patient presents with different clinical scenarios and laboratory profiles. In order to properly direct the diagnosis and antimicrobial treatment in sepsis and severe infections, pathogenesis must be confirmed, and the causative agent must be identified with blood culture.

The elderly, young children, and neonates, as well as immunosuppressed patients such as those using corticosteroids, antineoplastics, and other treatments, long-term diabetic patients, those with a history of major trauma and operations, vascular grafts, prostheses, and other medical devices, constitute special vulnerable groups for infectious processes. Healthcare workers should eliminate colonization risks, such as vascular catheterization, unnecessary vascular access, and urinary catheters, and remove them when not in use. Both diagnostic characteristics and investigations to be ordered differ from those of the general population in these groups. Additionally, principles of antimicrobial treatment will be tailored to the specific needs of these selected populations.

In patients with suspected severe infection, assessing and monitoring vital parameters, including consciousness, providing vascular access, should be routinely performed without delay in differential diagnosis after brief history taking and initial examination. All patients with signs and symptoms consistent with an infectious disease and physiological deterioration should be screened for sepsis. Sepsis is the most common cause of death in critical patients. The mortality rate of septic shock lies between 20% and 40% in developed countries, although it varies substantially from center to center. Sepsis is in the differential diagnosis of most serious conditions in the primary care and emergency setting, including anaphylaxis, acute coronary syndromes, hypovolemia, shock states, etc. Emergency recognition of sepsis and septic shock increases the survival of patients. Factors affecting poor outcomes in these patients suspected or diagnosed with sepsis include shock, hyperlactatemia, and organ failure. Atypical presentations should be emphasized in the training of triage and ED personnel due to difficulties and pitfalls in diagnostic processes for sepsis. Critical interventions such as lactate measurement, obtaining blood cultures, administration of fluid therapy, restoration of oxygenation, and appropriate antibiotic treatment compose the prerequisites for survival. Vasopressor support, rapid initiation of antimicrobials, and, in selected cases, glucocorticoids are mandatory in patients with septic shock.

The vital organ functions of the elderly, who are among the highest risk groups in the management of sepsis, may deteriorate rapidly with very few precursors, and aggressive methods should be used rapidly when necessary. Interactions of drug doses in the elderly, issues with excretion, and variations in metabolism should be taken into account when developing treatment regimens. In the long term, after recovery from sepsis, heart failure, peripheral vascular disease, dementia, and diabetes are the most common entities recorded in the literature.

Increasing public awareness of the issue, developing evidence-based measures, and management by healthcare professionals are essential in increasing survival.

The chain is as strong as its weakest link. Therefore, this book project aims to highlight current diagnostic and treatment approaches for sepsis and severe infections.

Ozgur Karcıoglu
Department of Emergency Medicine,
Istanbul Education and Research Hospital,
University of Health Sciences,
Istanbul, Türkiye

Canan Akman
Department of Emergency Medicine,
Canakkale Onsekiz Mart University,
Canakkale, Türkiye

Göksu Afacan Ozturk
Department of Emergency Medicine,
Istanbul Aydin University,
Kucukcekmece, Istanbul, Türkiye

Chapter 1

Introductory Chapter: The Infections of Humanity or the Humanity of Infections? What Will Save Us from the Era of Pandemics?

Canan Akman, Göksu Afacan Ozturk and Ozgur Karcıoglu

1. Overview

The history of infectious diseases is almost as old as human history. Throughout history, very few factors have influenced human life and development as much as infectious diseases and the microorganisms that cause them. Over the ages, epidemics have affected the population of societies by destroying hundreds of thousands and millions of people over months or years, destroying empires, changing the course of wars, and transforming human lifestyles.

The traumatic effects inflicted by the smallpox epidemic on the American continent and Indian culture have not healed for a long time. The plague ended feudalism in Medieval Europe, and the upheaval laid the seeds of the modern economic systems. Malaria led to certain improvements in the slave trade practices. Syphilis has led to some restrictions on sexual freedom. Nevertheless, a recent modelling study outlined that substantial gains in survival have occurred in every global region over the past 50 years [1]. The authors estimated that vaccination has accounted for 40% of the observed decline in global infant mortality, 52% in the African region.

The late medieval plague outbreak caused by *Yersinia pestis* is widely known as "The Black Death." This name represented the bubonic plague pandemic that emerged and reigned in Europe from 1346 to 1353 [2]. It was one of the most fatal pandemics in human history; as many as 50 million people were afflicted, paving the way to the loss of around half of Europe's fourteenth-century population [3].

Advances in medicine after the 1900s witnessed mankind's debatable victory over microscopic agents. Interestingly, in 1969, General W. Stewart, a surgeon, declared that the era of infectious diseases had ended in his speech in the U.S. Congress [4]. However, it has become clear how fake this victory is with the advent of the AIDS epidemic, not even 20 years later. Over these years, infections with AIDS, Ebola virus infection, Legionnaires' Disease, Mad Cow Disease, and bacteria strains that have become resistant to many antibiotics have gained importance. As a result, the attention of science circles, public opinion, and governments at the beginning of the twenty-first century has been concentrated on infectious diseases again, with the effect of the old fears. The 2009–2010 swine flu-H1N1 outbreaks

IntechOpen

have left deep traces in industrialized countries, the western world, and developing countries and introduced masks and disinfectants, and new vaccines to the large populations under threat.

2. How does a country defeat epidemics?

This is a difficult and multifactorial question. The prevalence of COVID-19 in neighboring countries, the intensity of the country's relationship with other countries, age, and other demographic factors affect the aggressiveness of the outbreak. Many additional factors, such as the virulence of the virus, the level of immunity of the population, vaccination, and minimization of damage through

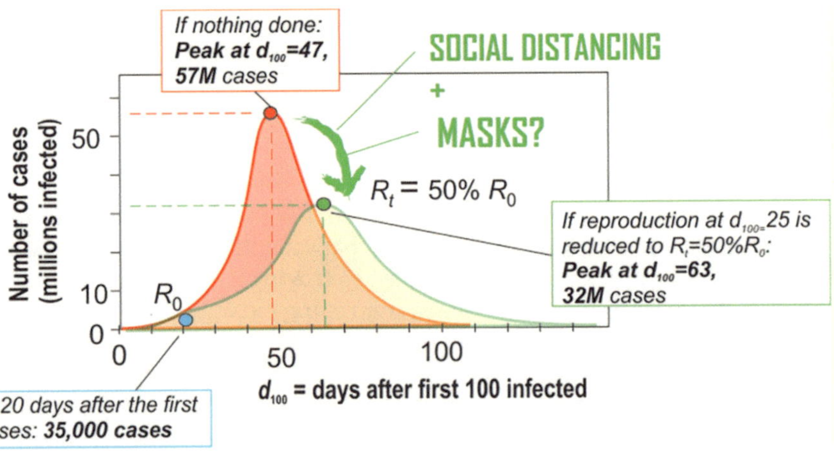

Figure 1.
With the intensive use of personal protective equipment and the imposition of individual isolation and social restrictions, the increments in the number of infected cases will be spread over time, and sudden loads on the health system will be tolerated more easily.

1. Virulence, that is, the measured ability of an infectious agent to infect human tissues, or the disease-causing ability associated with the severity of the disease it causes.
2. Identification of cases by testing multiple people, including asymptomatic ones.
3. Isolation: Isolating diagnosed and suspicious cases from healthy people.
4. Filing (filiation in French, used in most developing countries, including Turkey): To open a file for the diagnosed case and to examine it in detail with all the connections and contacts, to monitor their condition by phone or home visit, to ensure that they take their medication, and to ensure rapid intervention in the development of complications.
5. Contact person: Someone who has had an epidemiological relationship with the animal or environment that leads to the possibility of acquiring that infection.
6. Contact tracing: To identify and monitor individuals who have some contact with diagnosed and suspicious cases and to ensure that they are tested for identification.
7. Prevention of arrivals from abroad: To stop their arrival in the country by sea, land, and air or to allow their entry after certain procedures (such as quarantine).

Table 1.
Important terms in the management of pandemic periods include the glossary below.

drugs and healthcare institutions, will affect how much society is harmed by the disease (**Figure 1**). Tests for detecting cases, reporting systems (filing), and surveillance are effective factors concerning the state health organization's response to this disease. Other than these, factors affecting the country's struggle with the pandemic are listed in **Table 1**.

3. Pandemic and lessons learned

The outbreak of COVID-19 at the end of 2019 made humanity say, "nothing will be like before anymore," just like the 1918 flu pandemic (Spanish flu) and the 1957–1958 Asian flu pandemic that had radically changed the world in the previous century. As a result of the SARS-CoV-2 pandemic, we experienced dreadful times in which more than 7 million people were counted as "registered" deaths, while many victims were buried without even being counted officially in developing countries. In the pandemic that had started in China, a serious spread was seen primarily in European countries with dense populations (**Figure 2**). However, European countries, which reached expanded vaccination goals after 2021, were able to reduce the number of cases and deaths rapidly. Failure to achieve mass protection because of vaccine inequality in developing countries led to the death of hundreds of thousands of elderly and those with uncontrolled chronic diseases. Lack of democracy and equality contributed to the failure to explain the importance of vaccines to the target populations, and the inability to reach effective vaccines due to economic reasons increased losses, and most patients appear to die on class grounds.

While influenza outbreaks cause children, young, and productive-age people to face serious disease risk, COVID-19 poses a serious threat to the fragile malnourished

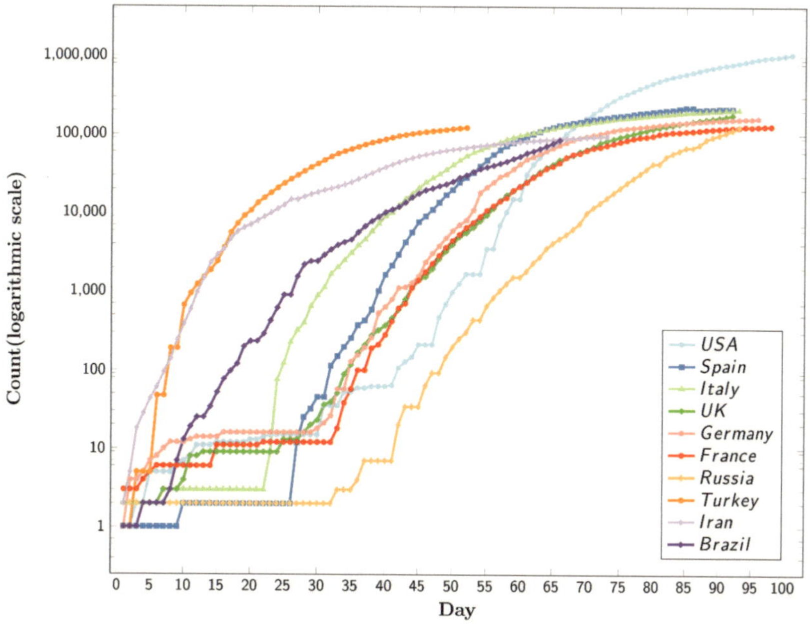

Figure 2.
Semi-logarithmic graph showing total cumulative case numbers of the 10 most affected countries from the date of the first case.

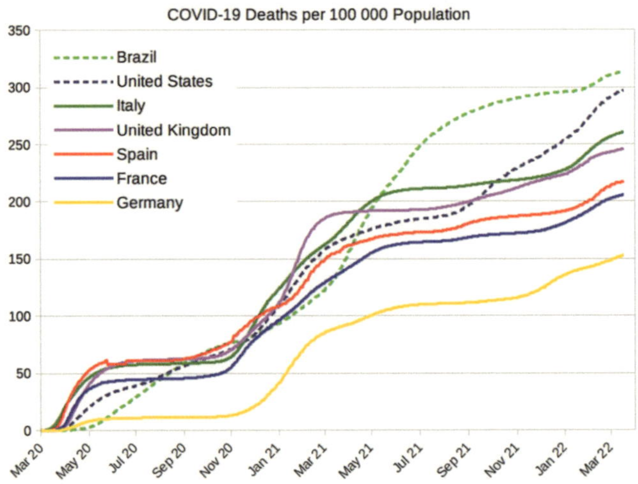

Figure 3.
There is a softer rise in the COVID-19 pandemic in European countries that have successfully implemented and maintained effective vaccination programs in 2021 after the initial rise in 2020. More serious and permanent rises were recorded in countries such as Brazil and the United States, where the health care system has been poorly organized, and vaccination cannot be carried out extensively due to various hesitations and health ignorance.

patients and those patients with poor health care due to poverty, and risks have emerged in our lives with coffins and tombstones instead of dry, soulless graphics.

Vaccines like Sinovac, developed by China, were not effective enough and did not pass scientific challenges (phase studies), becoming the dominant vaccine option in the lands where billions lived and leading to increased deaths with the prudent approval of world monopolist capitalism. The incidence and mortality rates in each country have been affected in relation to the effectiveness of vaccination campaigns **(Figure 3).** On May 5, 2023, the World Health Organization announced that the pandemic is no longer a global emergency.

The total (cumulative) number of COVID-19 cases in the world increased to 704 million, 7,010,000 of them dead (1% death rate) as of May 2025 [5]. Almost half of the cases are in five countries: The USA, Brazil, India, Russia, and Mexico. Of course, this information is unlikely to be entirely credible because countries have completely different ways of detecting a case or attributing a death to COVID-19. Especially China, the homeland of the pandemic, has scarcely yielded official and reliable data on its losses. Interestingly, China declared only around 5200 deaths officially.

The Delta virus spreads more easily and widely than the other strains. Since the virus attaches to human beings` ACE-2 receptors and enters cells using the spike (S) protein, the mutation of the Delta variant facilitates this attachment and enables us to "grab" the virus more easily from the air. Research has also revealed this. Incidentally, these ACE2 receptors, which we have always blamed, are more abundant in men, cardiac patients, and the elderly, which explains why the disease attacks older men more frequently.

The approach known as "mask, distancing, hygiene (MDH)" has been suggested to protect from the disease. Factors such as the period spent with the sick person, virus load, ventilation quality, and how many m^3 of air are available per person (the room volume) directly affect the transmission. If we add "time" and "ventilation" to the formula, the MDH + TV formula emerges instead of MDH. So, we will get used to thinking with more factors and taking precautions from now on. To explain this better, I would like to remind you that even if people chatting indoors in a guesthouse are masked, the longer the conversation, the more contagious it will be, and when you are in a crowded, unventilated, and dense environment, it will be very easy to get infected again.

Both the scientific community and the people of the world (and, of course, the rulers) should put their hats down and discuss how to eradicate the disease with the least damage by creating a participatory, democratic, well-founded scientific strategy, as well as preventing the next pandemic. In brief, we are on the last exit before the next pandemic.

Author details

Canan Akman[1], Göksu Afacan Ozturk[2] and Ozgur Karcıoglu[3]*

1 Department of Emergency Medicine, Canakkale Onsekiz Mart University, Canakkale, Turkey

2 Department of Emergency Medicine, Istanbul Aydin University, Kucukcekmece, Istanbul, Turkey

3 Department of Emergency Medicine, Istanbul Education and Research Hospital, University of Health Sciences, Istanbul, Turkey

*Address all correspondence to: okarcioglu@gmail.com

References

[1] Shattock AJ, Johnson HC, Sim SY, et al. Contribution of vaccination to improved survival and health: Modelling 50 years of the expanded programme on immunization. Lancet. 2024;**403**(10441):2307-2316. DOI: 10.1016/S0140-6736(24)00850-X

[2] Christakos G, Olea RA, Serre ML, Wang LL, Yu HL. Interdisciplinary Public Health Reasoning and Epidemic Modelling: The Case of Black Death. Berlin, Heidelberg: Springer; 2005. ISBN 978-3-540-25794-3.

[3] Mukharjee A. Economic Life after Covid-19: Lessons from the Black Death. The Economic Times.; 2020. Available from: https://economictimes.indiatimes.com/markets/stocks/news/economic-life-after-covid-19-lessons-from-the-black-death/articleshow/74870296.cms [Accessed: 2 May 2025]

[4] Spellberg B. Dr. William H. Stewart: Mistaken or maligned? Clinical Infectious Diseases. 2008;**47**(2):294. DOI: 10.1086/589579

[5] Coronavirus Tracker. Available from: https://www.worldometers.info/coronavirus/ [Accessed: 5 May 2025].

Chapter 2

Ventilator Management during Controlled and Triggered Breaths in ARDS Patients

Chang-Wen Chen

Abstract

Ventilatory therapy plays a critical role in managing patients with Acute Respiratory Distress Syndrome (ARDS). The primary goal of ventilator therapy is to assist in ventilation while preventing ventilator-induced lung injury (VILI) and ventilator-induced diaphragm dysfunction (VIDD). Volutrauma and atelectrauma are the main mechanisms responsible for VILI. Recently, respiratory rate and flow rate have been highlighted as possible elements contributing to VILI, and the concept of mechanical power was proposed. Once patients are able to breathe spontaneously, efforts should focus on avoiding patient self-inflicted lung injury (P-SILI). Prolonged paralysis of the diaphragm or patient-ventilator dyssynchrony can lead to VIDD or P-SILI. To achieve less injurious ventilation, careful selection of Positive End-Expiratory Pressure (PEEP) and tidal volume is crucial. However, determining the optimal ventilator settings remains a challenge, as it depends on the specific characteristics of each patient and the judgment of the physician. Therefore, critical care physicians should have a comprehensive understanding of the pathophysiological basis of ARDS and be aware of the current consensus regarding ventilator management for these patients.

Keywords: ARDS, recruitment, patient self-inflicted lung injury, pendelluft, atelectrauma

1. Introduction

Since Ashbaugh et al. [1] introduced the term 'acute respiratory distress in adults' to describe a condition characterized by acute onset of tachypnea, hypoxemia, and loss of compliance after a variety of stimuli in 12 patients, acute respiratory distress syndrome (ARDS) has become one of the cardinal illnesses in intensive care units. Mechanical ventilation is commonly used in patients with ARDS, and the definition of ARDS has evolved several times [2–4]. The 2012 Berlin definition, which classifies ARDS into three severity levels, became the prevalent classification [4]. For patients with moderate to severe ARDS, controlled mechanical ventilation, often coupled with deep sedation or even paralysis, may be necessary to achieve low tidal volume ventilation with positive end-expiratory pressure (PEEP) [5]. The selection of PEEP is a subject of ongoing debate [6]. Once patients are allowed to resume triggered breathing, ensuring appropriate breathing efforts becomes an important consideration. Both for controlled and triggered breathing, lung-and diaphragm-protective ventilation strategies need to be considered [7, 8]. The core mechanisms proposed for ventilator-induced lung injury (VILI) include atelectrauma [9, 10], volutrauma [11–13], and patient self-inflicted lung injury (P-SILI) [14, 15], all of which may lead to biotrauma [16]. Mechanisms of P-SILI included increased pulmonary transvascular pressure, pendelluft with focal lung overdistention, patient-ventilator dyssynchrony. In recent years, the role of respiratory and flow rates in lung injury has garnered attention from leading physiologists, and the concept of mechanical power was introduced [17–19]. This chapter will briefly review ventilator management for two different breathing statuses in ARDS patients, namely controlled and triggered breathing under mechanical ventilation, and will discuss individualized decisions regarding ventilator settings.

2. Modes of ventilation

Ventilators are used in one of two modes. In the controlled breathing mode, the ventilator settings control the ventilator's air volume, driving pressure, and frequency, with no input from the patient (**Figure 1a**). In triggered breathing mode, breath cues from the patient trigger the flow from the ventilator (**Figure 1b**). For both controlled and triggered breathing, lung- and diaphragm-protective ventilation strategies need to be considered.

a. Controlled breathing mode

In controlled breathing mode, the patient is completely relaxed and does not trigger the ventilator, and it is primarily used in patients with moderate to severe

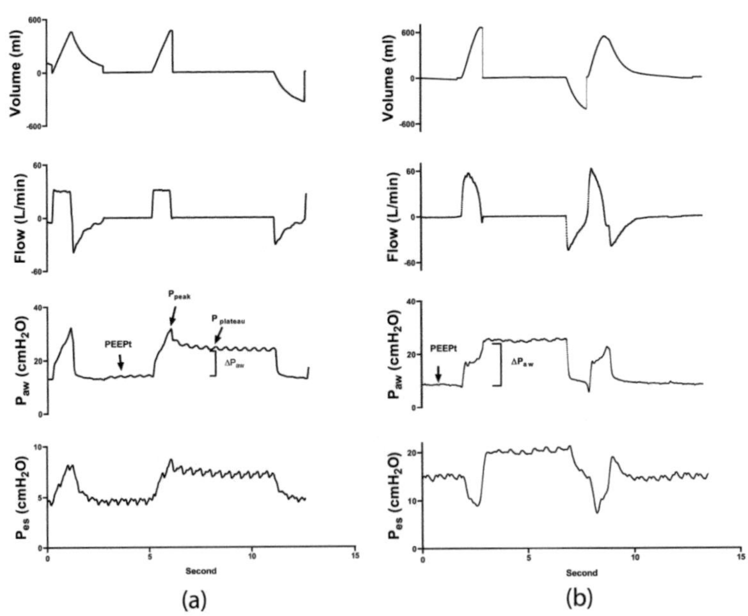

Figure 1.
Schematic description of constant flow control ventilation (a) and triggered pressure control ventilation with end-inspiratory occlusion (b). P_{aw}: airway pressure; P_{es}: esophageal pressure; P_{peak}: peak airway pressure. $P_{Plateau}$: airway plateau pressure; PEEPt: total PEEP. ΔP_{aw}: airway driving pressure. Respiratory system compliance = volume/ΔP_{aw} (ml/cmH$_2$O).

ARDS. Relaxation is often induced through sedation or even paralysis to achieve low tidal volume with PEEP [5]. Pressure control and volume control ventilation are two most frequently used controlled modes.

b. Triggered breathing mode

In triggered breathing mode, the ventilator is triggered by breath cues from the patient. Once patients are allowed to resume triggered breathing, ensuring appropriate breathing efforts becomes an important consideration. Various modes could be applied during triggered breathing [20].

3. Mechanisms of lung damage

a. Volutrauma and atelectrauma [11]

Alveolar overdistention (volutrauma) and intratidal opening and closure (atelectrauma) are two classical mechanisms of VILI. Inappropriate tidal volume or high PEEP may lead to alveolar overdistension, but intratidal lung opening and closure may occur if inappropriate PEEP is applied in patients with high recruitability. Atelectrauma is predominant in dependent/lower lung regions while volutrauma usually occurs in nondependent/upper lung regions [21].

b. Pulmonary edema caused by increased transvascular pressure

In cases of excessive spontaneous breathing effort, increased negative pleural pressure can lead to heightened transvascular pressure, exacerbating lung edema [22]. Negative pressure pulmonary edema is a recognized phenomenon [15, 22–24]. Once lung edema develops, lung volume decreases, further exacerbating lung injury.

c. Pendelluft in ARDS patients (**Figure 2**)

Pendelluft, or the air shift from nondependent to dependent lung regions, was first described by Yoshida et al. in a pig lung injury model [15]. The cause of pendelluft in injured lungs is related to heterogeneous pleural pressure distribution during breathing effort [15]. High levels of pendelluft can cause regional alveolar hyperinflation, even if low tidal volume is maintained. Pendelluft is believed to increase with breathing effort, but its degree varies among ARDS patients [26, 27]. Some patients may exhibit minimal pendelluft despite increasing breathing effort [26, 27]. Pendelluft is reported to increase in patients with focal ARDS or those with higher lung compliance [26]. However, the best method to quantify pendelluft in ventilated patients remains a matter of debate [25, 27, 28]. Furthermore, the mode of mechanical ventilation or patient-ventilator dyssynchrony can influence the severity of pendelluft. Pendelluft has been observed not only in trigger breaths but also in reverse triggering breaths [26, 29].

d. Patient-Ventilator dyssynchrony in ARDS Patients (**Figure 3**)

Patient-ventilator dyssynchrony is common in patients undergoing assisted mechanical ventilation [30]. About one-fourth of ICU patients exhibit a high

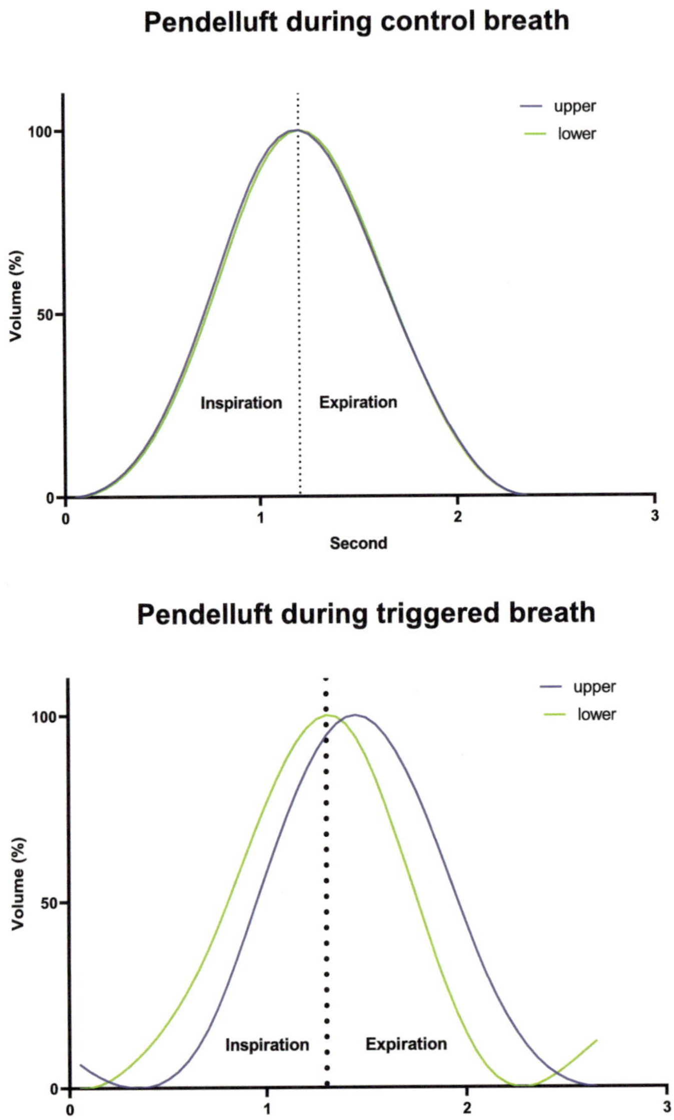

Figure 2.
A schematic representation of pendelluft measurement at rest and during triggered breathing shows a significant phase shift between the upper (nondependent) region and the lower (dependent) region. The y-axis represents the change in lung volume, normalized from 0 to 100% for the upper and lower lung regions, respectively. This method was proposed by Cornejo et al. [25].

incidence of major asynchronies, including ineffective triggering, double triggering, and autotriggering [31, 32]. A recent study revealed that minor dyssynchronies, such as early and late cycling and trigger delay, may be more frequent in patients under pressure support ventilation [33]. Reverse triggering was observed in 30–55% of sedated patients under controlled ventilation [34]. Some reverse-triggered breaths may be associated with breath stacking, which is a form of patient-ventilator dyssynchrony. In this condition, consecutive machine inspiratory cycles occur in close succession with incomplete exhalation between them, and it can lead to volutrauma if excessive tidal volume occurs [34, 35] and may result in diaphragm injury if excessive respiratory effort is used [36]. A high cumulative duration of clusters of double triggering in mechanically ventilated patients is associated with a longer ICU length of stay, fewer ventilator-free days,

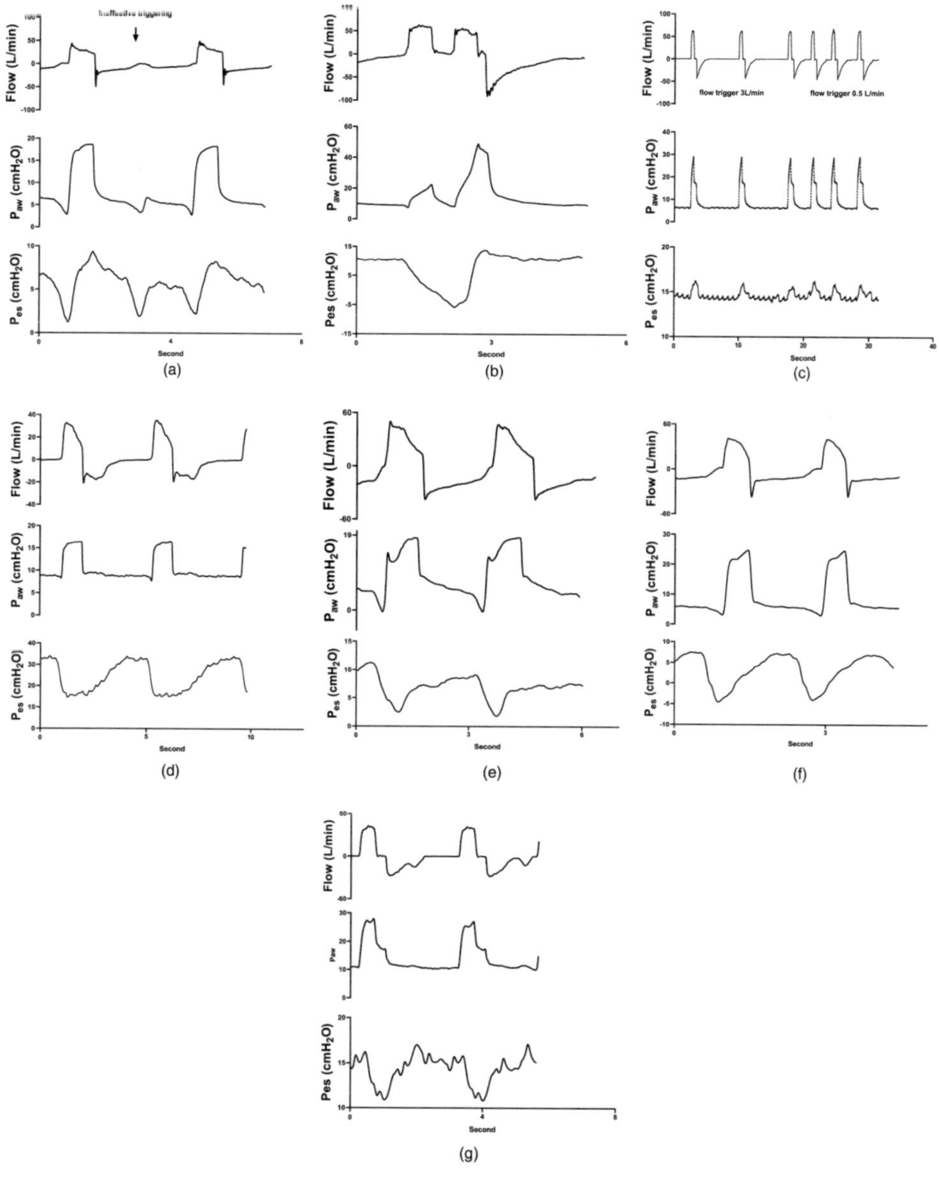

Figure 3.
a: Ineffective triggering was defined as an inspiratory effort (decrease in esophageal pressure of >1 cm H_2O) with a simultaneous drop in airway pressure, change in flow, or both; b: Double triggering was defined as two breath cycles separated by a very short expiratory time, specifically less than one-half of the mean inspiratory time; c: Autotriggering was defined as a cycle delivered by the ventilator without a decrease in esophageal pressure of >1 cm H_2O; d: Early cycling was defined as a machine inspiratory time shorter than the patient's inspiratory time by at least 250 ms; e: Late cycling was defined as a machine inspiratory time longer than the patient's inspiratory time by at least 250 ms; f: Trigger delay was defined as the time gap between the start of patient effort and machine delivery time being longer than 250 ms; g: Reverse triggering was defined as the ventilator delivering a breath that triggers respiratory efforts from the patient; P_{aw}: refers to airway pressure; P_{es}: esophageal pressure.

and shorter survival duration compared to patients with a low cumulative duration of clusters [37]. Expiratory muscle activity during triggered breathing may exert strong counter-effects to PEEP and resulted in decreased end-expiratory lung volume which may lead to hypoxemia or atelectrauma [26, 38].

4. Methods for PEEP and tidal volume decision

4.1 Selection of PEEP

PEEP is often selected based on PEEP/fraction of oxygen tables in various large clinical trials [39–42]. With a standard tidal volume of 6 ml per kilogram of predicted body weight and an airway plateau pressure limitation of less than 30 cmH_2O, Probabilities of survival and discharge at 60 days are similar whether lower or higher PEEP protocols are used [40]. Therefore, PEEP selection should ideally be based on objective, individualized measurements [43]. The chosen PEEP should achieve significant lung recruitment without causing overdistension.

4.2 Conventional methods for PEEP selection

Several conventional methods are used to determine PEEP. All of these methods can be implemented with some commercial ventilators that have appropriate embedded software.

1. *Pressure-volume curve*: This method uses the inspiratory or expiratory limb of the pressure-volume curve to identify the lower and higher inflection points for PEEP selection [44, 45]. Syringe, low flow or pressure ramp methods [44–46] can be used. Objective inflection points could be obtained with an optimization process of a sigmoidal equation (**Figure 4**) [47]. PEEP is set to 2 cmH2O above the inspiratory lower inflection point. However, the lung is usually not fully recruited at the lower inflection point plus 2 cmH2O. For the utility of the expiratory limb, PEEP is usually selected as the level at which oxygenation decreases, signifying alveolar collapse. Unfortunately, alveolar collapse (or derecruitment) is a continuous process that begins at high PEEP levels [48]. Therefore, it is difficult to determine the appropriate level of PEEP to select. Moreover, determining the optimal PEEP from the expiratory limb is challenging because this segment of the curve cannot discriminate regional ventilation distribution [49]. Therefore, the use of a single pressure-volume curve for PEEP selection is questionable.

2. *Stress Index (SI)*: This method uses the airway pressure-time profile to assess tidal recruitment or overdistension (**Figure 5**) [50–52]. Constant flow and volume-cycled ventilation must be employed, and appropriate segmentation, signal processing, and optimization processes are necessary to obtain the SI. During the constant flow inhalation period, the airway pressure (p_a) is modeled as a function of time (t) as

$$p_a = at^b + c$$

and the parameter b is defined as the stress index. A b value of 1 indicates a linear relationship. A b value greater than 1 indicates that the rate of change

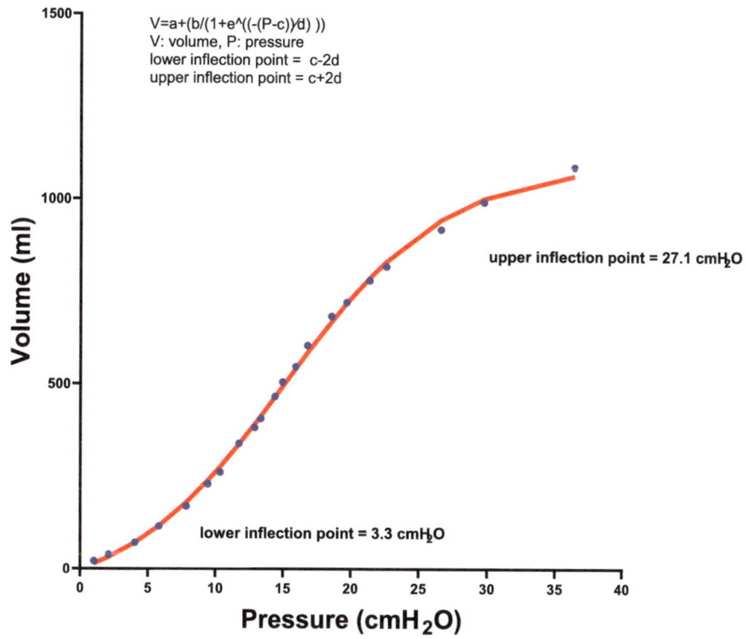

Figure 4.
Pressure-volume data from a patient fitted with the sigmoidal function proposed by Venegas et al. [47]. Blue dots represent the original data points, and the red line represents the fitted curve.

of pressure tends to increase with time (with volume) so that the lungs become more stiff as they fill. Conversely, $b < 1$ means that the slope decreases with time. A SI between 0.9 and 1.1 is considered acceptable [50, 52]. An SI less than 0.9 implicates tidal recruitment, and PEEP should be increased. On the other hand, an SI greater than 1.1 implicates overdistension, and PEEP should be decreased [52]. SI could be used in daily clinical practice if non-pulmonary factors influencing SI are taken into consideration [51]. But SI does not reflect regional ventilation heterogeneity.

3. *Best compliance*: This commonly used method involves selecting PEEP based on the best compliance following decremental PEEP titration. With an airway driving pressure (ΔPaw) of 15 cm H2O, PEEP is progressively increased up to 24 cm H2O. Then, PEEP is decreased from 24 to 6 cm H2O in steps of 2 cm H2O under volume control ventilation of 5 ml/kg predicted body weight [53]. Respiratory system compliance is calculated as tidal volume divided by ΔPaw. Typically, the PEEP associated with maximum compliance plus 2 cm H2O is selected. A recruitment maneuver using a higher airway pressure range and decremental PEEP titration was employed in an alveolar recruitment trial, which showed increased mortality in ARDS patients when PEEP selection was based on best compliance compared to patients with low PEEP [13]. Furthermore, it has been found that best compliance correlates poorly with recruitment volume [54], leading to controversy surrounding both the selection of best compliance and the use of recruitment maneuvers. Additionally, more than one PEEP value may show the best compliance (with a difference in compliance of less than 1 cm H2O between two PEEP levels). Information regarding regional ventilation distribution is crucial for selecting the appropriate PEEP in such scenarios [55].

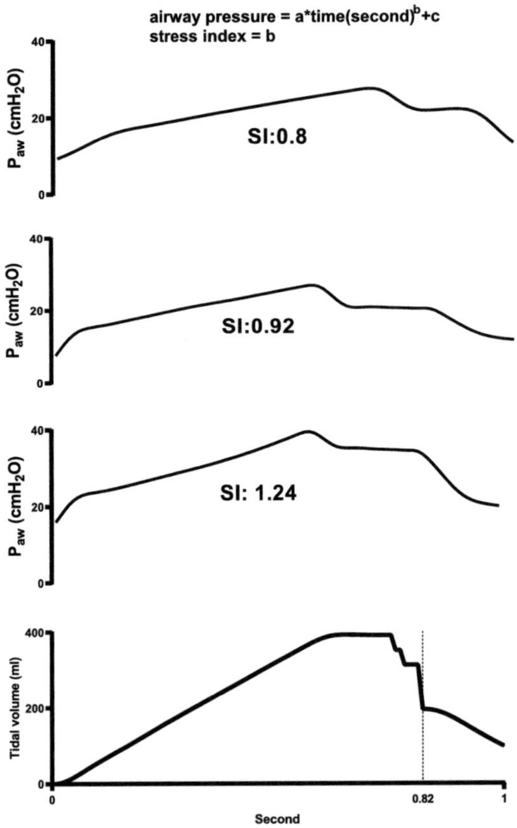

Figure 5.
The airway pressure-time profile during constant flow ventilation was fitted with the inserted power law equation, and the exponential coefficient calculated from this equation represents the stress index. Tidal volume-time profile is the case with SI of 1.24.

4.3 Novel methods for PEEP selection

The prevalent point of view in current medicine is personal and precise [56]. Different phenotypes of ARDS may respond differently to the PEEP strategy [57]. In addition, bedside recruitability to the level of PEEP applied is crucial for PEEP selection [58–60]. Unfortunately, the definition of lung recruitment depends on the method of measurement used [61]. Measurement of lung recruitment by computed tomography is regarded as the gold standard, but it cannot be used practically on a daily basis, unfortunately. Respiratory mechanics-based methods [60, 62, 63] and EIT-based method [64] are used at bedside. The criteria of high or low recruiter remains disputed.

1. *Recruitment-to-inflation ratio*: To simplify the measurement of recruitment volume, Dellamonica et al. [60] initially used the difference in end-expiratory lung volume (EELV) between two PEEP levels and the minimal predicted increase in lung volume to calculate the recruitment volume between high and low PEEP. In order to afford clinical usefulness, Chen et al. [62] proposed a single-breath method to quantify the recruited volume which could be implanted on the ventilator directly. Following a decrease in PEEP from 15 to 5 cmH_2O, the recruited volume at a PEEP of 15 cmH_2O could be estimated by subtracting the minimal

change in lung volume from PEEP 15 to 5 cmH_2O (specifically, the respiratory system compliance at a PEEP of 5 cmH_2O multiplied by the PEEP change). The recruitment compliance was calculated as the recruited volume divided by the difference in PEEP or by the difference between the high PEEP and airway opening pressure (when airway opening pressure is higher than low PEEP). The recruitment to inflation ratio is simply the ratio between recruitment compliance and compliance at low PEEP [63]. A recruitment-to-inflation ratio of zero would indicate lack of recruitment. High and low recruiters are distinguished based on the recruitment-to-inflation ratio. They define a recruitment-to-inflation ratio greater than 0.5 as indicative of a high recruiter. Since its publication, the recruitment-to-inflation ratio has gained popularity. However, determining the exact PEEP level remains challenging because the relationship between recruitment volume and PEEP levels is non-linear [62, 63]. Recruitability is not uniform, and a parabolic behavior between the recruitment-to-inflation ratio and PEEP from 0 to 15 cmH_2O is observed in most patients with ARDS, making it challenging to determine the appropriate PEEP level to be selected [63].

2. *Tidal lung hysteresis*: Mojoli et al. [65] designed a new approach by combining consideration of the low-flow pressure-volume loop and respiratory system compliance. Tidal hysteresis was quantified as the area enclosed by the pressure-volume loop, normalized by the change in pressure (thus having units of mL). The PEEP level was selected as the PEEP level associated with a small change in tidal hysteresis (<10 mL/cmH_2O between sequential PEEP levels). In cases where several PEEP levels exhibited small changes in tidal hysteresis, the PEEP with the highest respiratory system compliance was selected. This approach revealed a significant difference in PEEP selection between high tidal recruiters and biphasic recruiters, which exhibit a small increase in hysteresis at high PEEP and a large increase in hysteresis below a certain PEEP, compared to low tidal recruiters. They found that tidal hysteresis ≥100 mL is highly predictive of tidal recruitment at the next PEEP step reduction. Lung hysteresis is related to tidal recruitment, as observed from chest CT scans [66]. Selection of PEEP based on lung hysteresis may prevent atelectrauma. Understandably, the PEEP level selected is significantly higher when lung hysteresis is taken into consideration in high tidal recruiters [65]. The viewpoint that PEEP is selected according to lung hysteresis and respiratory system compliance is attractive because tidal recruitment-derecruitment could be minimized, while overdistension could also be lessened.

3. *Electrical Impedance Tomography (EIT):* EIT is increasingly used in ICUs for PEEP titration, with several methods based on different criteria [67–73]. EIT is characterized by its low spatial resolution (similar to scintigraphy) but high temporal resolution. It reveals regional ventilation distribution during mechanical ventilation, where PEEP application creates different distributions in dependent and nondependent regions.

EIT measures the impedances between multiple electrodes placed around the chest. In a manner similar to computer aided tomography, these measurements are converted from impedance as a function of surface location to impedance as a function of location within the chest volume. Because air has a much larger impedance than tissue, well-inflated regions are identified in the impedance map as high impedance locations. The volume measurements are combined with the ventilator pressure to compute a

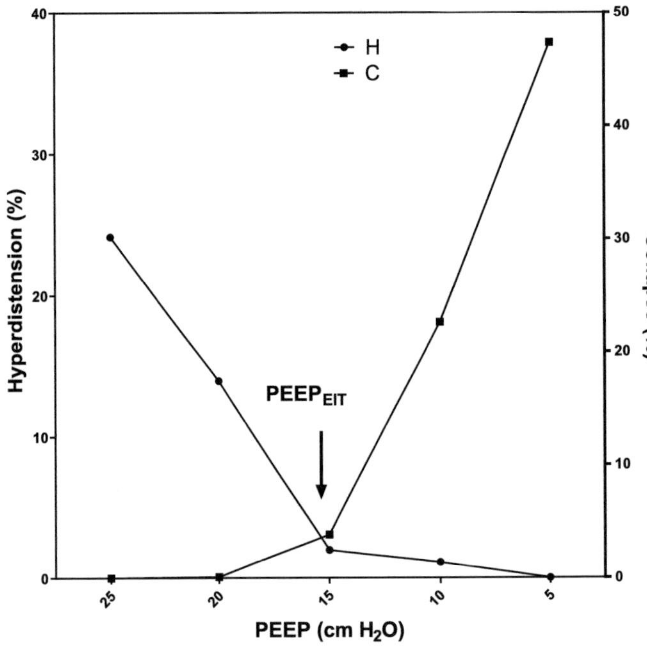

Figure 6.
Graphic representation of the crossover point between the collapse (C) and hyperdistension (H) curves and the corresponding PEEP level. PEEP$_{EIT}$: PEEP selected according to the crossing point.

spatial map of compliance. Regions of the lung with decreased compliance during high pressure are considered to be overdistended, while regions that demonstrate decreased compliance at low pressure are considered to be collapsed. The percent areas that are overdistended and collapsed are then plotted as a function of PEEP (**Figure 6**).

The most common approach is to select the PEEP level at the intersection of the overdistension-collapse curve, aiming to balance recruitability and overdistension [53, 68]. Between the lowest and highest PEEP levels, the proportion of collapse and hyperdistension can be calculated based on changes in regional compliance at each PEEP level. Lung overdistension and collapse coexist during decremental PEEP titration, and the PEEP level at the crossing point of the overdistension-collapse curve is assumed to be appropriate for selection [68]. In the recent RECRUIT trial [53], conducted in COVID-19 ARDS patients, PEEP settings were personalized considering recruitability and overdistension. The low and medium recruitability groups had a higher PEEP at the crossing point compared to the PEEP associated with the highest compliance, whereas no difference was found in the highly recruitable group. The PEEP selected using these two methods differed in 80% of cases. However, the advantages of this method compared to others remain to be determined.

4.3.1 Tidal volume selection

Since the milestone ARDSNet study [39], low tidal volume ventilation (6 ml/Kg IBW) with preselected PEEP based on fraction of inspired oxygen (FiO_2) usage has become the standard for ARDS patients [39–42]. In 2015, Amato proposed the concept of targeting airway driving pressure instead of low tidal volume in adjusting tidal volume because lung stress, instead of tidal volume, was a determinant of VILI.

Maintaining an airway driving pressure below 15 cmH_2O is an appropriate target for ARDS patients [74, 75]. Mortality was positively correlated with both driving pressure and respiratory rate in retrospective analyses of pooled data from clinical trials [76]. In cases with high elastance, tidal volume could be lower than 6 ml/Kg, with a higher respiratory rate allowed. In contrast, in cases with low elastance, a higher tidal volume may be permissible with lower respiratory rate [76].

4.3.1.1 Practical ventilatory management of controlled ventilation

Although both atelectrauma and volutrauma are important in VILI, priority should be given to avoiding alveolar overdistension, as suggested by recent clinical studies [13, 77]. If regional ventilation distribution is not available at the bedside, selection of PEEP with the lowest driving pressure and preselected low tidal volume should be considered. The recruitment-to-inflation ratio, measurable at the bedside, can guide PEEP adjustment; in high recruiters (e.g., recruitment-to-inflation ratio >1), higher PEEP may be applied. Additionally, high PEEP is advisable in obese ARDS patients and those with chest wall abnormalities [78]. In these cases, measuring esophageal pressure to assess transpulmonary pressure may be necessary. Once esophageal pressure is established, titrating PEEP to maintain end-expiratory transpulmonary pressure between −2 and 2 cmH_2O is recommended [79]. For tidal volume selection, patients with low respiratory system elastance (<25 cmH_2O/L) may be allowed a higher range of tidal volume than those with high elastance (>25 cmH_2O/L). If no further information is available, initial PEEP settings of 5–10, 10–15, 15–20 cmH_2O corresponding to mild, moderate, and severe degrees of ARDS can be used [49], with adjustments following to maintain airway driving pressure below 15 cmH_2O.

4.3.1.2 Practical ventilatory management during triggered breath

For mechanically ventilated ARDS patients, triggered breaths are permissible if good patient-ventilator interaction is observed and tidal volume is within expected limits. Although maintaining a driving pressure below 15 cmH_2O is ideal, accurately estimating this pressure in spontaneously breathing patients can be challenging [80–82]. In these patients, excessive respiratory effort should be avoided due to its adverse effects, which include increased negative pleural pressure potentially exacerbating lung edema, decreased end-expiratory lung volume leading to intratidal opening and closing of alveoli, and acceleration of the pendelluft phenomenon [22]. Additionally, patient-ventilator dyssynchrony may further compromise respiratory muscles or lung function [22].

Although targeting low tidal volume or low airway driving pressure remains important during triggered breaths, achieving these targets can be challenging. Adequate sedation and analgesics, appropriate ventilator settings, and regular monitoring of breathing effort, are essential [83–85]. Studies have shown that breathing effort can be estimated, but only for extremes of effort [84]. In cases of persistent excessive breathing effort, the placement of esophageal pressure monitoring or titrating dose of neuromuscular blocking agent to allow weaker effort may be indicated [86, 87]. The goals for target volume and airway driving pressure are the same as for controlled breaths. Regular end-expiratory occlusion maneuvers [85], including both occlusion and negative pressure measurements, should provide invaluable information to clinicians. Respiratory muscle pressure (Pm) and dynamic transpulmonary pressure ($\Delta P_{L,dyn}$) can be assessed using a brief expiratory occlusion. The optimal

Pm is between 5 to 10 cmH_2O, and it is advisable to keep Pm below 15 cmH_2O. $\Delta P_{L,dyn}$ should be less than 20 cmH_2O [85]. While excessive respiratory effort, often caused by inadequate ventilator assistance, is undesirable, overassistance from the ventilator, leading to excessively low respiratory effort, is also not ideal.

5. Conclusions

Many studies have been conducted since the inaugural study of low tidal volume ventilation in ARDS patients by Amato et al. [88]. The standard of ventilatory support is evolving [89]. Current standards include limiting driving pressure to <15 cmH2O and adjusting the respiratory rate to minimize the mechanical power of breathing. PEEP selection remains undecided. However, ventilatory support is just one part of managing ARDS patients. Ventilation adjuncts such as prone ventilation and extra-corporeal membrane oxygenation (ECMO) are used in moderate to severe cases [89]. Some pharmacotherapy may also be beneficial for ARDS patients [89]. Critical care physicians should constantly stay updated with the latest consensus on managing ARDS patients.

Author details

Chang-Wen Chen[1,2]

1 Section of Critical Care Medicine and Section of Pulmonary Medicine, Department of Internal Medicine, National Cheng Kung University Hospital, Tainan, Taiwan

2 Department of Medicine, College of Medicine, National Cheng Kung University, Tainan, Taiwan

*Address all correspondence to: cwchen@mail.ncku.edu.tw

References

[1] Ashbaugh DG, Bigelow DB, Petty TL, Levine BE. Acute respiratory distress in adults. Lancet. 1967;**2**(7511):319-323

[2] Murray JF, Matthay MA, Luce JM, Flick MR. An expanded definition of the adult respiratory distress syndrome. The American Review of Respiratory Disease. 1988;**138**(3):720-723

[3] Bernard GR, Artigas A, Brigham KL, Carlet J, Falke K, Hudson L, et al. Report of the American-European consensus conference on acute respiratory distress syndrome: Definitions, mechanisms, relevant outcomes, and clinical trial coordination. Consensus Committee. Journal of Critical Care. 1994;**9**(1):72-81

[4] Force ADT, Ranieri VM, Rubenfeld GD, Thompson BT, Ferguson ND, Caldwell E, et al. Acute respiratory distress syndrome: The Berlin definition. JAMA. 2012;**307**(23):2526-2533

[5] Alhazzani W, Belley-Cote E, Moller MH, Angus DC, Papazian L, Arabi YM, et al. Neuromuscular blockade in patients with ARDS: A rapid practice guideline. Intensive Care Medicine. 2020;**46**(11):1977-1986

[6] Gattinoni L, Marini JJ. In search of the holy grail: Identifying the best PEEP in ventilated patients. Intensive Care Medicine. 2022;**48**(6):728-731

[7] Goligher EC, Dres M, Patel BK, Sahetya SK, Beitler JR, Telias I, et al. Lung- and diaphragm-protective ventilation. American Journal of Respiratory and Critical Care Medicine. 2020;**202**(7):950-961

[8] Chiumello D, Dres M, Camporota L. Lung and diaphragm protective ventilation guided by the esophageal pressure. Intensive Care Medicine. 2022;**48**(10):1302-1304

[9] Tremblay L, Valenza F, Ribeiro SP, Li J, Slutsky AS. Injurious ventilatory strategies increase cytokines and c-fos m-RNA expression in an isolated rat lung model. The Journal of Clinical Investigation. 1997;**99**(5):944-952

[10] Muscedere JG, Mullen JB, Gan K, Slutsky AS. Tidal ventilation at low airway pressures can augment lung injury. American Journal of Respiratory and Critical Care Medicine. 1994;**149**(5):1327-1334

[11] Guldner A, Braune A, Ball L, Silva PL, Samary C, Insorsi A, et al. Comparative effects of volutrauma and atelectrauma on lung inflammation in experimental acute respiratory distress syndrome. Critical Care Medicine. 2016;**44**(9):e854-e865

[12] Bellani G, Guerra L, Musch G, Zanella A, Patroniti N, Mauri T, et al. Lung regional metabolic activity and gas volume changes induced by tidal ventilation in patients with acute lung injury. American Journal of Respiratory and Critical Care Medicine. 2011;**183**(9):1193-1199

[13] Writing Group for the Alveolar Recruitment for Acute Respiratory Distress Syndrome Trial I, Cavalcanti AB, Suzumura EA, Laranjeira LN, Paisani DM, Damiani LP, et al. Effect of lung recruitment and titrated positive end-expiratory pressure (PEEP) vs low PEEP on mortality in patients with acute respiratory distress syndrome: A randomized clinical trial. JAMA. 2017;**318**(14):1335-1345

[14] Brochard L, Slutsky A, Pesenti A. Mechanical ventilation to minimize progression of lung injury in acute respiratory failure. American Journal of Respiratory and Critical Care Medicine. 2017;**195**(4):438-442

[15] Yoshida T, Torsani V, Gomes S, De Santis RR, Beraldo MA, Costa EL, et al. Spontaneous effort causes occult pendelluft during mechanical ventilation. American Journal of Respiratory and Critical Care Medicine. 2013;**188**(12):1420-1427

[16] Slutsky AS, Ranieri VM. Ventilator-induced lung injury. The New England Journal of Medicine. 2013;**369**(22):2126-2136

[17] Marini JJ, Rocco PRM, Gattinoni L. Static and dynamic contributors to ventilator-induced lung injury in clinical practice. Pressure, energy, and power. American Journal of Respiratory and Critical Care Medicine. 2020;**201**(7):767-774

[18] Gattinoni L, Collino F, Camporota L. Mechanical power: Meaning, uses and limitations. Intensive Care Medicine. 2023;**49**(4):465-467

[19] Gattinoni L, Tonetti T, Cressoni M, Cadringher P, Herrmann P, Moerer O, et al. Ventilator-related causes of lung injury: The mechanical power. Intensive Care Medicine. 2016;**42**(10):1567-1575

[20] Mireles-Cabodevila E, Siuba MT, Chatburn RL. A taxonomy for patient-ventilator interactions and a method to read ventilator waveforms. Respiratory Care. 2022;**67**(1):129-148

[21] Caironi P, Cressoni M, Chiumello D, Ranieri M, Quintel M, Russo SG, et al. Lung opening and closing during ventilation of acute respiratory distress syndrome. American Journal of Respiratory and Critical Care Medicine. 2010;**181**(6):578-586

[22] Yoshida T, Fujino Y, Amato MB, Kavanagh BP. Fifty years of research in ARDS. Spontaneous breathing during mechanical ventilation. Risks, mechanisms, and management. American Journal of Respiratory and Critical Care Medicine. 2017;**195**(8):985-992

[23] Bhaskar B, Fraser JF. Negative pressure pulmonary edema revisited: Pathophysiology and review of management. Saudi Journal of Anaesthesia. 2011;**5**(3):308-313

[24] Roshdy A, Katira BH, Kuebler WM, Kavanagh BP. Vascular-induced lung injury: Another advocate for personalized ARDS management: Discussion on "inspiratory preload obliteration may injure lungs via cyclical 'on-off' vascular flow". Intensive Care Medicine. 2018;**44**(4):540-541

[25] Cornejo RA, Arellano DH, Ruiz-Rudolph P, Guinez DV, Morais CCA, Gajardo AIJ, et al. Inflammatory biomarkers and pendelluft magnitude in ards patients transitioning from controlled to partial support ventilation. Scientific Reports. 2022;**12**(1):20233

[26] Lin WC, Su PF, Chen CW. Pendelluft in patients with acute respiratory distress syndrome during trigger and reverse triggering breaths. Scientific Reports. 2023;**13**(1):22143

[27] Coppadoro A, Grassi A, Giovannoni C, Rabboni F, Eronia N, Bronco A, et al. Occurrence of pendelluft under pressure support ventilation in patients who failed a spontaneous breathing trial: An observational study. Annals of Intensive Care. 2020;**10**(1):39

[28] Sang L, Zhao Z, Yun PJ, Frerichs I, Moller K, Fu F, et al. Qualitative and

quantitative assessment of pendelluft: A simple method based on electrical impedance tomography. Annals of Translational Medicine. 2020;**8**(19):1216

[29] Yoshida T, Nakamura MAM, Morais CCA, Amato MBP, Kavanagh BP. Reverse triggering causes an injurious inflation pattern during mechanical ventilation. American Journal of Respiratory and Critical Care Medicine. 2018;**198**(8):1096-1099

[30] Murias G, Lucangelo U, Blanch L. Patient-ventilator asynchrony. Current Opinion in Critical Care. 2016;**22**(1):53-59

[31] Thille AW, Rodriguez P, Cabello B, Lellouche F, Brochard L. Patient-ventilator asynchrony during assisted mechanical ventilation. Intensive Care Medicine. 2006;**32**(10):1515-1522

[32] Chen CW, Lin WC, Hsu CH, Cheng KS, Lo CS. Detecting ineffective triggering in the expiratory phase in mechanically ventilated patients based on airway flow and pressure deflection: Feasibility of using a computer algorithm. Critical Care Medicine. 2008;**36**(2):455-461

[33] Mojoli F, Pozzi M, Orlando A, Bianchi IM, Arisi E, Iotti GA, et al. Timing of inspiratory muscle activity detected from airway pressure and flow during pressure support ventilation: The waveform method. Critical Care. 2022;**26**(1):32

[34] Rodrigues A, Telias I, Damiani LF, Brochard L. Reverse triggering during controlled ventilation: From physiology to clinical management. American Journal of Respiratory and Critical Care Medicine. 2023;**207**(5):533-543

[35] Beitler JR, Sands SA, Loring SH, Owens RL, Malhotra A, Spragg RG, et al. Quantifying unintended exposure to high tidal volumes from breath stacking dyssynchrony in ARDS: The BREATHE criteria. Intensive Care Medicine. 2016;**42**(9):1427-1436

[36] Damiani LF, Engelberts D, Bastia L, Osada K, Katira BH, Otulakowski G, et al. Impact of reverse triggering dyssynchrony during lung-protective ventilation on diaphragm function: An experimental model. American Journal of Respiratory and Critical Care Medicine. 2022;**205**(6):663-673

[37] Sousa M, Magrans R, Hayashi FK, Blanch L, Kacmarek RM, Ferreira JC. Clusters of double triggering impact clinical outcomes: Insights from the EPIdemiology of patient-ventilator aSYNChrony (EPISYNC) cohort study. Critical Care Medicine. 2021;**49**(9):1460-1469

[38] Plens GM, Droghi MT, Alcala GC, Pereira SM, Wawrzeniak IC, Victorino JA, et al. Expiratory muscle activity counteracts positive end-expiratory pressure and is associated with fentanyl dose in patients with acute respiratory distress syndrome. American Journal of Respiratory and Critical Care Medicine. 2024;**209**(5):563-572

[39] Acute Respiratory Distress Syndrome N, Brower RG, Matthay MA, Morris A, Schoenfeld D, Thompson BT, et al. Ventilation with lower tidal volumes as compared with traditional tidal volumes for acute lung injury and the acute respiratory distress syndrome. The New England Journal of Medicine. 2000;**342**(18):1301-1308

[40] Brower RG, Lanken PN, MacIntyre N, Matthay MA, Morris A, Ancukiewicz M, et al. Higher versus lower positive end-expiratory pressures in patients with the acute respiratory distress syndrome. The New England Journal of Medicine. 2004;**351**(4):327-336

[41] Meade MO, Cook DJ, Guyatt GH, Slutsky AS, Arabi YM, Cooper DJ, et al. Ventilation strategy using low tidal volumes, recruitment maneuvers, and high positive end-expiratory pressure for acute lung injury and acute respiratory distress syndrome: A randomized controlled trial. JAMA. 2008;**299**(6):637-645

[42] Mercat A, Richard JC, Vielle B, Jaber S, Osman D, Diehl JL, et al. Positive end-expiratory pressure setting in adults with acute lung injury and acute respiratory distress syndrome: A randomized controlled trial. JAMA. 2008;**299**(6):646-655

[43] Gattinoni L, Collino F, Camporota L. Assessing lung recruitability: Does it help with PEEP settings? Intensive Care Medicine. 2024;**50**(5):749-751

[44] Jonson B. Elastic pressure-volume curves in acute lung injury and acute respiratory distress syndrome. Intensive Care Medicine. 2005;**31**(2):205-212

[45] Gattinoni L, Pesenti A, Avalli L, Rossi F, Bombino M. Pressure-volume curve of total respiratory system in acute respiratory failure. Computed tomographic scan study. The American Review of Respiratory Disease. 1987;**136**(3):730-736

[46] Demory D, Arnal JM, Wysocki M, Donati S, Granier I, Corno G, et al. Recruitability of the lung estimated by the pressure volume curve hysteresis in ARDS patients. Intensive Care Medicine. 2008;**34**(11):2019-2025

[47] Venegas JG, Harris RS. Simon BA: A comprehensive equation for the pulmonary pressure-volume curve. Journal of Applied Physiology. 1985/1998;**84**(1):389-395

[48] Crotti S, Mascheroni D, Caironi P, Pelosi P, Ronzoni G, Mondino M, et al. Recruitment and derecruitment during acute respiratory failure: A clinical study. American Journal of Respiratory and Critical Care Medicine. 2001;**164**(1):131-140

[49] Gattinoni L, Carlesso E, Cressoni M. Selecting the 'right' positive end-expiratory pressure level. Current Opinion in Critical Care. 2015;**21**(1):50-57

[50] Grasso S, Terragni P, Mascia L, Fanelli V, Quintel M, Herrmann P, et al. Airway pressure-time curve profile (stress index) detects tidal recruitment/hyperinflation in experimental acute lung injury. Critical Care Medicine. 2004;**32**(4):1018-1027

[51] Formenti P, Graf J, Santos A, Gard KE, Faltesek K, Adams AB, et al. Non-pulmonary factors strongly influence the stress index. Intensive Care Medicine. 2011;**37**(4):594-600

[52] Terragni P, Bussone G, Mascia L. Dynamic airway pressure-time curve profile (stress index): A systematic review. Minerva Anestesiologica. 2016;**82**(1):58-68

[53] Jonkman AH, Alcala GC, Pavlovsky B, Roca O, Spadaro S, Scaramuzzo G, et al. Lung recruitment assessed by electrical impedance tomography (RECRUIT): A multicenter study of COVID-19 acute respiratory distress syndrome. American Journal of Respiratory and Critical Care Medicine. 2023;**208**(1):25-38

[54] Su PL, Lin WC, Ko YF, Su PF, Chen CW. Positive end-expiratory pressure selection based on best respiratory system compliance or collapse/hyperdistension curves in patients with acute respiratory distress syndrome: Lack of correlation with alveolar recruitment. Intensive Care Medicine. 2018;**44**(3):389-391

[55] Su PL, Lin WC, Ko YF, Cheng KS, Chen CW. Electrical impedance tomography analysis between two similar respiratory system compliance during decremetal PEEP titration in ARDS patients. Journal of Medical and Biological Engineering. 2021;**41**(6):888-894

[56] Beitler JR, Thompson BT, Baron RM, Bastarache JA, Denlinger LC, Esserman L, et al. Advancing precision medicine for acute respiratory distress syndrome. The Lancet Respiratory Medicine. 2022;**10**(1):107-120

[57] Calfee CS, Delucchi K, Parsons PE, Thompson BT, Ware LB, Matthay MA, et al. Subphenotypes in acute respiratory distress syndrome: Latent class analysis of data from two randomised controlled trials. The Lancet Respiratory Medicine. 2014;**2**(8):611-620

[58] Amato MB, Santiago RR. The recruitability paradox. American Journal of Respiratory and Critical Care Medicine. 2016;**193**(11):1192-1195

[59] Gattinoni L, Marini JJ, Quintel M. Recruiting the acutely injured lung: How and why? American Journal of Respiratory and Critical Care Medicine. 2020;**201**(2):130-132

[60] Dellamonica J, Lerolle N, Sargentini C, Beduneau G, Di Marco F, Mercat A, et al. PEEP-induced changes in lung volume in acute respiratory distress syndrome. Two methods to estimate alveolar recruitment. Intensive Care Medicine. 2011;**37**(10):1595-1604

[61] Chiumello D, Marino A, Brioni M, Cigada I, Menga F, Colombo A, et al. Lung recruitment assessed by respiratory mechanics and computed tomography in patients with acute respiratory distress syndrome. What is the relationship? American Journal of Respiratory and Critical Care Medicine. 2016;**193**(11):1254-1263

[62] Chen L, Del Sorbo L, Grieco DL, Junhasavasdikul D, Rittayamai N, Soliman I, et al. Potential for lung recruitment estimated by the recruitment-to-inflation ratio in acute respiratory distress syndrome. A clinical trial. American Journal of Respiratory and Critical Care Medicine. 2020;**201**(2):178-187

[63] Grieco DL, Pintaudi G, Bongiovanni F, Anzellotti GM, Menga LS, Cesarano M, et al. Recruitment-to-inflation ratio assessed through sequential end-expiratory lung volume measurement in acute respiratory distress syndrome. Anesthesiology. 2023;**139**(6):801-814

[64] Mauri T, Eronia N, Turrini C, Battistini M, Grasselli G, Rona R, et al. Bedside assessment of the effects of positive end-expiratory pressure on lung inflation and recruitment by the helium dilution technique and electrical impedance tomography. Intensive Care Medicine. 2016;**42**(10):1576-1587

[65] Mojoli F, Pozzi M, Arisi E, Mongodi S, Orlando A, Maggio G, et al. Tidal lung hysteresis to interpret PEEP-induced changes in compliance in ARDS patients. Critical Care. 2023;**27**(1):233

[66] Chiumello D, Arnal JM, Umbrello M, Cammaroto A, Formenti P, Mistraletti G, et al. Hysteresis and lung recruitment in acute respiratory distress syndrome patients: A CT scan study. Critical Care Medicine. 2020;**48**(10):1494-1502

[67] Wrigge H, Zinserling J, Muders T, Varelmann D, Gunther U, von der Groeben C, et al. Electrical impedance tomography compared with thoracic computed tomography during a slow inflation maneuver in experimental

models of lung injury. Critical Care Medicine. 2008;**36**(3):903-909

[68] Costa EL, Borges JB, Melo A, Suarez-Sipmann F, Toufen C Jr, Bohm SH, et al. Bedside estimation of recruitable alveolar collapse and hyperdistension by electrical impedance tomography. Intensive Care Medicine. 2009;**35**(6):1132-1137

[69] Lowhagen K, Lundin S, Stenqvist O. Regional intratidal gas distribution in acute lung injury and acute respiratory distress syndrome assessed by electric impedance tomography. Minerva Anestesiologica. 2010;**76**(12):1024-1035

[70] Liu S, Tan L, Moller K, Frerichs I, Yu T, Liu L, et al. Identification of regional overdistension, recruitment and cyclic alveolar collapse with electrical impedance tomography in an experimental ARDS model. Critical Care. 2016;**20**(1):119

[71] Spadaro S, Mauri T, Bohm SH, Scaramuzzo G, Turrini C, Waldmann AD, et al. Variation of poorly ventilated lung units (silent spaces) measured by electrical impedance tomography to dynamically assess recruitment. Critical Care. 2018;**22**(1):26

[72] Nestler C, Simon P, Petroff D, Hammermuller S, Kamrath D, Wolf S, et al. Individualized positive end-expiratory pressure in obese patients during general anaesthesia: A randomized controlled clinical trial using electrical impedance tomography. British Journal of Anaesthesia. 2017;**119**(6):1194-1205

[73] Eronia N, Mauri T, Maffezzini E, Gatti S, Bronco A, Alban L, et al. Bedside selection of positive end-expiratory pressure by electrical impedance tomography in hypoxemic patients: A feasibility study. Annals of Intensive Care. 2017;7(1):76

[74] Amato MB, Meade MO, Slutsky AS, Brochard L, Costa EL, Schoenfeld DA, et al. Driving pressure and survival in the acute respiratory distress syndrome. The New England Journal of Medicine. 2015;**372**(8):747-755

[75] Roca O, Goligher EC, Amato MBP. Driving pressure: Applying the concept at the bedside. Intensive Care Medicine. 2023;**49**(8):991-995

[76] Costa ELV, Slutsky AS, Brochard LJ, Brower R, Serpa-Neto A, Cavalcanti AB, et al. Ventilatory variables and mechanical power in patients with acute respiratory distress syndrome. American Journal of Respiratory and Critical Care Medicine. 2021;**204**(3):303-311

[77] Cressoni M, Chiumello D, Algieri I, Brioni M, Chiurazzi C, Colombo A, et al. Opening pressures and atelectrauma in acute respiratory distress syndrome. Intensive Care Medicine. 2017;**43**(5):603-611

[78] Heunks L, Piquilloud L, Demoule A. How we approach titrating PEEP in patients with acute hypoxemic failure. Critical Care. 2023;**27**(1):415

[79] Sarge T, Baedorf-Kassis E, Banner-Goodspeed V, Novack V, Loring SH, Gong MN, et al. Group EP-S: Effect of esophageal pressure-guided positive end-expiratory pressure on survival from acute respiratory distress syndrome: A risk-based and mechanistic reanalysis of the EPVent-2 trial. American Journal of Respiratory and Critical Care Medicine. 2021;**204**(10):1153-1163

[80] Bertoni M, Spadaro S, Goligher EC. Monitoring patient respiratory effort during mechanical ventilation: Lung and diaphragm-protective ventilation. Critical Care. 2020;**24**(1):106

[81] Soundoulounaki S, Akoumianaki E, Kondili E, Pediaditis E, Prinianakis G,

Vaporidi K, et al. Airway pressure morphology and respiratory muscle activity during end-inspiratory occlusions in pressure support ventilation. Critical Care. 2020;**24**(1):467

[82] Bellani G, Grassi A, Sosio S, Foti G. Plateau and driving pressure in the presence of spontaneous breathing. Intensive Care Medicine. 2019;**45**(1):97-98

[83] Bertoni M, Telias I, Urner M, Long M, Del Sorbo L, Fan E, et al. A novel non-invasive method to detect excessively high respiratory effort and dynamic transpulmonary driving pressure during mechanical ventilation. Critical Care. 2019;**23**(1):346

[84] de Vries HJ, Tuinman PR, Jonkman AH, Liu L, Qiu H, Girbes ARJ, et al. Performance of noninvasive airway occlusion maneuvers to assess lung stress and diaphragm effort in mechanically ventilated critically ill patients. Anesthesiology. 2023;**138**(3):274-288

[85] Dianti J, Bertoni M, Goligher EC. Monitoring patient-ventilator interaction by an end-expiratory occlusion maneuver. Intensive Care Medicine. 2020;**46**(12):2338-2341

[86] Mauri T, Yoshida T, Bellani G, Goligher EC, Carteaux G, Rittayamai N, et al. Esophageal and transpulmonary pressure in the clinical setting: Meaning, usefulness and perspectives. Intensive Care Medicine. 2016;**42**(9):1360-1373

[87] Doorduin J, Nollet JL, Roesthuis LH, van Hees HW, Brochard LJ, Sinderby CA, et al. Partial neuromuscular blockade during partial ventilatory support in sedated patients with high tidal volumes. American Journal of Respiratory and Critical Care Medicine. 2017;**195**(8):1033-1042

[88] Amato MB, Barbas CS, Medeiros DM, Schettino Gde P, Lorenzi Filho G, Kairalla RA, et al. Beneficial effects of the "open lung approach" with low distending pressures in acute respiratory distress syndrome. A prospective randomized study on mechanical ventilation. American Journal of Respiratory and Critical Care Medicine. 1995;**152**(6 Pt 1):1835-1846

[89] Menk M, Estenssoro E, Sahetya SK, Neto AS, Sinha P, Slutsky AS, et al. Current and evolving standards of care for patients with ARDS. Intensive Care Medicine. 2020;**46**(12):2157-2167

Chapter 3

Bacterial Pneumonia in the Immunosuppressed Patient: An Update on Recognition and Management

Canan Akman, Göksu Afacan Ozturk, Feride Sinem Akgun, Bilgen Ozkaya and Ozgur Karcıoglu

Abstract

Cellular and humoral immune impairments develop following a disruption in systemic defense, which can be primary or acquired. Infectious and non-infectious lung problems may develop in immunosuppressed patients (ISP). Pneumonia is frequently seen in patients whose local or systemic defense mechanisms are impaired for any reason. In addition to treating lung diseases, the correct management of comorbid and underlying diseases is essential in these patients. A thorough understanding of the importance of bacterial pneumonia in ISP will be valuable for the correct diagnosis and management. *Pseudomonas aeruginosa* is a gram-negative bacterial agent that causes nosocomial pneumonia and various infections in ISP, as well as in those with structural lung disease. Preventive measures, including vaccination practices against viruses and Streptococcal disease, impacted the morbidity and mortality. This chapter aimed to systematically summarize and review current data on the diagnosis and management of pneumonia and related processes in ISP.

Keywords: pneumonia, bacterial pneumonia, immunosuppressed patient, immune suppression, lung infection, respiratory tract

1. Introduction

Cellular and humoral immune impairments develop as a result of disruption in systemic defense, which can be primary or acquired. Infectious and non-infectious lung problems may develop in immunosuppressed patients (ISP).

Pneumonia has long been an important trigger of mortality and disease states. Risk factors include young age, malnutrition, immunosuppression, tobacco smoke, or air pollution exposure. This infectious process is frequently seen in patients whose local or systemic defense mechanisms are impaired for any reason. In recent decades, advanced tools to obtain specimens and molecular techniques have caused improvements in microbiological diagnostics, which prove that lung infections stem from interactions of various microorganisms with each other. Reasons such as the subtle and atypical nature of clinical and laboratory findings, the co-existence of infectious and non-infectious problems, infection with polymicrobial agents, and the patient's inability to undergo diagnostic procedures render the recognition of pneumonia difficult and delayed in ISP. A basic microbiological workup should be performed in all ISPs who are hospitalized and in outpatients as well [1]. In the ISP, it is a priority to determine the type of immunodeficiency and to estimate the infectious agent accordingly and empirically.

In addition to the treatment of lung diseases, the correct management of comorbid and underlying diseases is essential for these patients. This chapter aimed to systematically summarize and review current data on the recognition and management of pneumonia and related processes.

2. Community-acquired pneumonia (CAP)

Community-acquired pneumonia (CAP) is the most common cause of mortality in pediatric patients below 5 years of age worldwide, although the optimal management of CAP in children remains to be elucidated. Currently, respiratory viruses are considered the most frequent agents. The death toll due to pneumonia has been reduced in children, although substantial and preventable numbers remain. Highly efficient interventions should be put into practice, and new strategies need to be developed [2]. Recent findings suggested that dual viral-bacterial infections (DVBI) had their synergistic impact on most patients and thus increased the severity of CAP. Brands and colleagues disclosed that CAP appears to be a shared property of immunocompromised status in septic individuals [3].

The co-existence of immune suppression and hyperinflammation in the case of CAP is considered an argument to refute the theory that there are two discrete stages during the host response to septic process. Hence, new and advanced technologies should be used to distinguish viral, bacterial, and DVBI from each other. Some authors proposed an efficient treatment strategy by searching for molecular pathogens, while transcriptome profiling will allow expedient and targeted therapies, paving the way for improved clinical courses in pediatric patients with CAP [4].

3. Decision aids for CAP in the immunosuppressed patient

Algorithms and decision aids have not been validated and should not be used for ISP or recently discharged patients [5]. For instance, patients may not be appropriate for outpatient treatment if they are unable to receive oral antibiotics or if they have significant psychosocial comorbidities. Physician clinical judgment may identify patients who warrant admission due to factors beyond those addressed by these aids. The PSI and CURB-65 must be used in conjunction with clinical judgment to assist in identifying patients for whom outpatient care may be considered if the treating physician identifies no other significant barriers to treatment. Patients receiving low-risk scores may be eligible for hospitalization in the presence of immune suppression, weakness in the respiratory muscles, dementia, serious psychiatric conditions, housing problems, or other comorbid medical or psychosocial conditions [6].

4. Complications in the immunosuppressed patients

Various complications can ensue in ISP involving the respiratory system, including lungs (**Table 1**). Bacterial, viral, and fungal pneumonia, TBC, and NTM infections constitute the majority.

Infectious complications	Non-infectious complications
I. Bacterial infections:	• Neoplastic problems (Kaposi's sarcoma, lymphoma)
• Staphylococcus aureus	
• Gram-negative (−) bacilli	• Pulmonary metastatic calcifications
• Legionella	• Lung damage due to drugs or radiation
• Listeria	• Hepatopulmonary syndrome
• Nocardia	• Pulmonary hypertension
• Pseudomonas aeruginosa	• Bronchiolitis obliterans
• Acinetobacter	• Diffuse alveolar hemorrhage
• Stenotrophomonas maltophilia	• Acute respiratory distress syndrome
• Haemophilus influenzae	• Pulmonary involvement of the primary disease
• Streptococcus pneumoniae	• Nonspecific interstitial pneumonia
• II. Mycobacterial infections:	
• Tuberculosis	
• Non-tuberculosis mycobacteriae	
III. Viral infections:	
• Cytomegalovirus	
• Respiratory viruses	
o İnfluenza	
o Parainfluenza	
o Adenovirus	
o Respiratory syncytial virus	
• Herpes zoster	
• Varicella zoster	
IV. Fungal infections:	
• Aspergillus	
• Pneumocystis jirovecii (carinii)	
• Candida	
• Other fungal infections	
• Cryptococcus neoformans	
• Zygomyçetes (esp. Mucor spp.)	
• Geographically endemic fungi (Histoplasma capsulatum, Coccidioides immitis, Blastomyces dermatitidis)	
• Scedosporium apiospermum	

Table 1.
Pulmonary complications in immunosuppressed patients.

4.1 Bacterial pneumonia in immunosuppressed patients

The incidence of ISP is rising due to new treatments in the fields of oncology, hematology, and transplantation, as well as longer life expectancy. These patients are at high risk of ICU follow-up due to the high rate of adverse outcomes. Severe CAP and resultant acute respiratory failure are among the most common factors for admission to hospital and ICU.

Among the infectious complications in ISP, bacterial pneumonia, which develops as CAP or nosocomial pneumonia (NP), is the most common entity. Severe pneumonia is inflicted by numerous pathogens. While bacterial pneumonia constitutes one-third of cases, viral and fungal pneumonia both compose up to 15% of cases. This specific group of patients needs invasive mechanical ventilation in high rates (up to 60%), associated with an in-hospital death rate of 40–50% [7]. Risk factors for septic shock following bacterial pneumonia include bacteremia, advanced age, and early infancy, uncontrolled diabetes mellitus, cancer, immunosuppressive states, and recent invasive procedures.

The relation between the intensity of the conditioning regimen and febrile neutropenia (FN), as well as their association with severe bacterial infections are yet to be elucidated. Facchini et al. analyzed the risk factors for FN and severe infections in 195 consecutive recipients of a reduced-intensity conditioning (RIC) allogeneic HSCT [8]. The RIC regimens consisted of fludarabine plus melphalan or busulfan, while severe bacterial infections included pneumonia, urinary tract infections, and bacteremia. After RIC-allo, FN and severe bacterial infections were identified mostly in patients with severe mucosal inflammation and early-onset neutropenia. In these patients, high-dose steroids given for acute GVHD were the prominent risk factor following engraftment procedure.

Pneumonia is among the most common adverse outcomes in both solid organ and HSCT. Clinical symptoms may appear late during infections in ISP. Clinicians should employ a more proactive approach with early recognition and a low threshold for empiric therapy [9]. The isolation of a pathogen in an upper airway sample does not always indicate the agent as the culprit in pneumonia. On the other hand, viral causes, including CMV, may coexist and contribute to opportunistic infections in transplant recipients. **Table 2** summarizes the relationship between patient risk factors and the specific agents inflicting pneumonia in ISP.

III.D. 1. Pneumococci are typical colonizers of ISP and a leading cause of CAP worldwide [10]. The percentages of patients afflicted by *S. pneumoniae* and *Haemophilus influenzae* type B have been reduced after the introduction of newly developed conjugate vaccines. *S. aureus* and *H. influenzae* non-type B are the commonly isolated bacteria, while viruses remain the most prevalent pathogenic agents [2]. The place and time of onset, causative pathogen, and clinical course are important in distinguishing between these two major types of pneumonia. Gram-negative bacteria and methicillin-resistant *S. aureus* (MRSA), and *Legionella* species are predominant in NP. *H. influenzae*, *S. pneumoniae*, and *Legionella* species are the most frequently isolated pathogens in patients diagnosed with CAP. Immunoglobulin (Ig) deficiency boosts the risk of infection via bacterial agents, especially *H. influenzae* and *S. pneumoniae*.

III.D. 2. P. aeruginosa is a gram-negative bacterium that causes nosocomial pneumonia and various infections in ISP, as well as in those with structural lung disease [11]. It is also one of the causative agents of ventilator-associated pneumonia, chronic infections in patients with cystic fibrosis, and bloodstream infections (BSI) in ISP [12].

Type of agent	Pathogens	Patient risk factors/conditions
Bacterial	*Streptococcus pneumoniae*	General immunosuppression, especially HIV/AIDS, hematologic malignancies, and organ transplantation
	Haemophilus influenzae	Splenic dysfunction, hypogammaglobulinemia, and respiratory diseases, such as COPD
	Staphylococcus aureus (including MRSA)	Prolonged hospital stays, indwelling catheters, and chronic steroids
	Gram-negative *Bacilli*, *P. aeruginosa*, *Klebsiella pneumonia*, and *Escherichia coli*	Neutropenia, prolonged hospitalization, mechanical ventilation, and broad-spectrum antibiotics
	Atypical bacteria, *Mycoplasma pneumonia*, *Legionella* species, *Chlamydia pneumoniae*	Milder immunosuppression and community-acquired infections
Viral	Cytomegalovirus (CMV)	Transplant recipients, HIV/AIDS
	Influenza virus	All immunosuppressed patients; high morbidity and mortality
	Respiratory Syncytial Virus (RSV)	Pediatric patients, transplant recipients
	Herpes Simplex Virus (HSV)	Severe immunodeficiency
	Varicella-zoster virus (VZV)	Hematologic malignancies, post-transplant conditions
Fungal	*Pneumocystis jirovecii*	HIV/AIDS, chronic immunosuppression
	Aspergillus species	Neutropenia, high-dose steroids
	Cryptococcus neoformans	HIV/AIDS
	Histoplasma capsulatum	Endemic areas, severe immunosuppression
	Coccidioides species	Endemic areas (southwestern USA), severe immunosuppression
Atypical Mycobacteria	Mycobacterium tuberculosis	HIV/AIDS, general immunosuppression
	Nontuberculous mycobacteria (NTM), Mycobacterium avium complex (MAC)	Advanced HIV/AIDS, chronic lung diseases

Table 2.
A summary of the key bacterial, viral, fungal, and atypical mycobacterial agents that cause pneumonia in immunosuppressed patients, along with the associated risk factors and conditions for each pathogen.

P. aeruginosa exhibits several virulence factors and various mechanisms of antibacterial resistance which played their role in increasing rates of antibacterial resistance in recent years [13]. Bloodstream infections (BSI) due to *P. aeruginosa* is associated with high complication and death rates, estimated between 43 and 59% [14–16]. Multi-drug resistant (MDR) BSIs caused by *P. aeruginosa* infection occur in 16.7–28% of cases and are associated with increased mortality [15, 16].

Interestingly, some lifestyle changes affect the incidence of certain infections in the ISP. For example, the COVID-19 pandemic triggered a boost in pet adoption, which caused more frequent contact of vulnerable people with these strains of bacteria [17].

III.D. 3. *Bordetella bronchiseptica* is among these opportunistic bacteria causing life-threatening infections in patients with HIV/AIDS. Animal exposure history was reported in 73% of the verified cases in a literature review by Gujju et al. [18]. The infection is characterized as an atypical pneumonia with persistent cough. Most commonly, *B. bronchiseptica* infection can be manifested with interstitial infiltrates accompanied by reduced CD4 lymphocyte counts in patients with HIV/AIDS. In some cases, it can cause severe sepsis and mortality. Immune suppression and chronic illnesses, including alcoholism, diabetes, and renal failure, are implicated in patients without HIV infection for contracting *B. bronchiseptica* infection. The most common infection site for P. aeruginosa is respiratory system, and it is the most commonly isolated gram-negative microorganism in NP, with an increasing prevalence in the past decades [19, 20].

III.D.4. *Corynebacterium striatum* has been reported in pulmonary infections, mostly as a conditioned pathogen in ISP, especially in patients with chronic structural lung diseases, paving the way for severe pneumonia, exacerbation of the underlying diseases, and increased death rate [21]. In addition, surgical or invasive procedures, prolonged hospital stays, advanced age, neoplastic disease, organ transplantation, HIV positivity, diabetes, antibiotic usage, and operations necessitating long-term use of devices—such as catheterization, heart valve implantation, and prosthesis—along with chronic diseases, long ICU stays, and anemia are known risk factors associated with *C. striatum* infection [22, 23]. In the post-pandemic era of COVID-19, the infection rate of *C. striatum* in the lower respiratory tract has markedly increased [24]. The agent exhibits MDR; therefore, vancomycin is considered the most effective treatment for C. striatum [21].

III.D.5. Gram-negative diplococci, including *Moraxella catarrhalis,* cause pneumonia in patients with preexisting lung disease, advanced age, treatment with corticosteroids, or other immunosuppressives. Pleural effusions and bacteremia are known complications in the involved patients.

Pneumocystis jirovecii pneumonia is encountered in the setting of AIDS, immunosuppressive or cytotoxic drug therapy, and cancer. Pneumothorax, respiratory failure, acute respiratory distress syndrome (ARDS), and fatal outcomes can be expected.

The evolution of hosts and bacteria gets along with each other simultaneously and interdependently. Hosts struggle with microbes that have developed various ways to avoid dying. *P. aeruginosa* infection gains persistence depending on the survival of the bacteria through the immune response. *P. aeruginosa* can achieve modulation of the host's immunity. The host immune system and bacteria coevolve, and our understanding of how bacteria overcome the immune response in ISPs is incomplete [25]. After binding to an epithelial cell, the type III secretion system of P. aeruginosa may be activated, which allows secretion of effector proteins into the epithelial cells, leading to cellular death [26].

Different mechanisms can play roles in immune suppression. Burn injuries constitute a typical example that cause significant systemic immune dysregulation and, later, immunosuppression. This immunosuppression resulting from burns renders patients susceptible to pulmonary and systemic colonization with nosocomial and opportunistic bacteria [27]. In a full-thickness burn model in rodents, Kartchner et al. indicated that burn-injured mice were less effective at clearing bacteria than sham-injured mice. Secondary infection is characterized by the migration of neutrophils and macrophages to the respiratory tract. These exhibited diminished secretion of antibacterial reactive O2 and nitrogen species and the pro-inflammatory cytokine IL-12, while macrophages showed increased release of the anti-inflammatory cytokines. Repeated infection leads to increased numbers of neutrophils and macrophages in lung tissues after burn injury, decreased immune functions, and enhanced expression of anti-inflammatory cytokines.

The microorganism invades pulmonary epithelia using its pili and flagella, and uses biofilm formation, quorum sensing, and a type III secretion mechanism to boost virulence [11].

4.2 Role of bronchoscopy and bronchoalveolar lavage (BAL) in ISP

Decisions regarding advanced investigations and more extensive workup, including bronchoscopy for BAL and/or bronchial biopsy, must be established on a case-by-case basis, considering risk factors for opportunistic pathogens [1].

In a systematic review, Gonski et al. pointed out that BAL helped diagnose a potential pathogen in 43% of cases in the evaluation of pulmonary lesions in children with ISP, while changing patient management after BAL was reported in more than half (53%) of cases [28]. Adverse events were generally mild, with no procedure-related mortality. The authors have postulated that BAL can be useful for assessing pulmonary disease in immunosuppressed children with reasonable safety.

While some pulmonary disorders have a highly characteristic signature of BAL findings, BAL results are mostly devoid of specificity and need to be interpreted along with other clinical and radiographic variables [29]. Various strains produce different accuracy rates in diagnostic processes. *B. bronchiseptica* was most commonly isolated from respiratory secretions, including bronchoalveolar lavage specimens [18].

Management of pulmonary complications after hematopoietic stem cell transplantation (HSCT) mostly encompasses bronchoalveolar lavage (BAL), but the diagnostic value of the procedure remains to be clarified in children who have undergone HSCT. Kasow et al. analyzed 78 allogeneic and 11 autologous transplant recipients who underwent BAL at a median of 68 days and 23 days after HSCT, respectively [30]. The most common indications for BAL in both populations were fever, hypoxia, and auscultatory findings. The most common finding was bacterial infection in both allogeneic and autologous patients (both around 60–70%). In summary, the safety and diagnostic yield of BAL is relatively high in children, but the likelihood of distinctive findings is lowered in allogeneic recipients with grade II–IV aGVHD and those receiving immunosuppressive treatment.

4.3 Antibiotic use in ISP

Advancing age is one of the factors contributing to immunosuppression, as it is mostly associated with organ failures and reduced physiological reserve. Antibiotic treatment for CAP in the elderly is particularly challenging for many reasons, including compliance, immunosuppression, and polypharmacy. Amalakuhan et al. launched the 'San Antonio NIPS model', aiming to reorganize clinicians' focus on antibiotic choices in the elderly that may have increasing importance in the future [31]. They identified seven novel antibiotics (solithromycin, pristinamycin, nemonaxacin, lefamulin, omadacycline, ceftobiprole, and delafloxacin) that currently promise effective utilization for the treatment of CAP in the elderly. All these compounds can be used efficiently in the elderly, but to varying degrees based on their NIPS model score. *B. bronchiseptica* can be treated with antipseudomonal penicillins combined with beta-lactamases, carbapenems, and fluoroquinolones [18].

Outpatient management for CAP in ISP is recommended for patients with comorbid medical conditions, such as chronic diseases involving the cardiovascular or pulmonary systems, liver, or kidney; uncontrolled diabetes; alcohol-related disorders; malignancies; post-splenectomy; immunocompromised states or use of immunosuppressant medications; or antibiotic use within 3 months.

a. Macrolide or doxycycline and a beta-lactam (amoxicillin/ clavulanate, cefpodoxime, or cefuroxime, twice daily).

b. Monotherapy with an oral fluoroquinolone (moxifloxacin, 400 mg daily; gemifloxacin, 320 mg daily; or levofloxacin, 750 mg daily).

Antibiotic use in patients with viral RTI is an issue worth debating. In a study including patients without secondary bacterial RTIs (mostly elderly), three-fourths were prescribed antibiotic treatment [32]. Beta-lactamase-sensitive penicillins and cephalosporins are among the agents most commonly ordered in these secondary bacterial RTIs. Patients receiving appropriate initial antibiotic therapy were shown to have lower incidences of treatment failure, shorter hospital costs, reduced death rates compared with patients who received inappropriate initial antibiotics [33].

MERINO study is a prospective randomized trial conducted to compare piperacillin-tazobactam with meropenem in ceftriaxone-resistant gram-negative bacteria, which are treated with a carbapenem [34]. The authors reported that noninferiority could not be established for piperacillin-tazobactam compared to meropenem, with 12.3% of the patients randomized to piperacillin-tazobactam dying within 30 days, compared to (3.7%) randomized to meropenem. **Table 3** indicates specific antibiotic and dosing recommendations for *P. aeruginosa* pneumonia.

Allo-SCT can result in long-term remission in patients with multiple myeloma (MM). Bensinger et al. reported that lenalidomide for relapsed MM after Allo-SCT may lead to prolonged disease control (>12 months) in half of the patients [35].

4.4 Statins used for treatment

Most research has demonstrated a reduced risk of CAP or a decrease in death rates due to CAP for current users of statins, but the observational designs of these research render the interpretation of their findings difficult. In a systematic review, Troeman et al. cited that statins alleviated pulmonary inflammatory processes by modulating neutrophil function, hampering cytokine expression, and protecting against disruption of pulmonary integrity [36].

4.5 Resistant cases to specific antimicrobial agents

In a systematic review, Ho et al. evaluated the evidence for the efficacy of screening, isolation, and decolonization of patients colonized or inflicted with vancomycin-resistant enterococci (VRE) and extended spectrum beta-lactamases-producing organisms in acute and long-term care facilities [37]. The presence and colonization of VRE and ESBL-producing microorganisms in the GI tract do not generally cause harm, but they may function as an infectious source in certain subgroups, such as ISP, physically debilitated, or those who underwent GI surgery. These hosts may also function as a reservoir for the transmission of VRE and ESBL-producing organisms to others.

Recently launched antibiotics against MDR *P. aeruginosa* have been shown to be clinically effective in the management of MDR *Pseudomonas* [11] (**Table 3**).

One of the regimens below	
Ceftazidime	IV 2 g tid or bid
Cefepime	IV 1–2 g tid
Piperacillin-tazobactam	IV 4.5 g qid
Meropenem	IV 2 g tid
Imipenem	IV 500 mg qid or 1 g tid
Aztreonam	IV 2 g tid
Plus (one of these)	
Tobramycin	IV 7 mg/kg od
Gentamicin	IV 7 mg/kg od
Levofloxacin	IV or PO 750 mg od
Ciprofloxacin	IV or PO 400 mg od
Amikacin	IV 20 mg/kg od
Antimicrobials for MDR-*P. aeruginosa* pneumonia	
Ceftolozane-tazobactam	IV 3 g tid
Ceftazidime-avibactam	IV 2.5 g tid
Imipenem-cilastatin-relebactam	IV 1.25 g qid
Cefiderocol	IV 2 g tid or qid

IV intravenous, MDR multi-drug resistant,
qid q 6 h tid q8 h od once daily.

Table 3.
Initial treatment of P. aeruginosa *pneumonia (for patients with normal renal and hepatic functions).*

Carbapenem: Recent years have witnessed an increase in the nosocomial infections caused by carbapenem-resistant *Klebsiella pneumoniae* (CRKP). Immunosuppressed states, ICU admission, antibiotic treatment (via carbapenems, quinolones, glycopeptides, and beta-lactamases/inhibitors), surgical interventions, mechanical ventilation, central venous catheterization, and nasogastric tubes are considered risk factors for CRKP infection in routine practice [38]. The main risk factors for carbapenem-resistant Enterobacterales (CRE) infections were found to be previous colonization, urinary catheter, and exposure to broad-spectrum antibiotics [39].

Penicillin: The increase in penicillin resistance over the years renders the treatment of these infections even more difficult. Gram-negative pathogens in neutropenic patients, *S. aureus* in cases with indwelling catheters, *Nocardia* in patients using long-term steroids, atypical agents, *H. influenza*, *S. pneumoniae* in cases with HIV—all of the bacteria listed above may be the cause of pneumonia, depending on whether they were acquired from the hospital or the community.

4.6 Preventive measures of pneumonia to be employed in the immunosuppressed patients

These are of utmost importance, since treatment of pneumonia would be more challenging in this vulnerable patient group, including life-threatening complications, such as ARDS and respiratory failure. **Table 4** provides a summary of preventive

Pneumonia etiology	Mode of prevention
Pneumococcal pneumonia	Pneumococcal vaccine
Influenza	Annual influenza vaccination; prophylaxis with oseltamivir in unvaccinated cases if there is an ongoing epidemic
Tuberculosis	Isoniazid prophylaxis
Cryptococcus neoformans	Fluconazole and conventional Amphotericin B
Pneumocystis pneumonia	Trimethoprim-sulfamethoxazole prophylaxis
Cytomegalovirus	Ganciclovir prophylaxis, preemptive therapy, receiving blood product from seronegative donor
Legionella	Control of water supplies and air conditioners
Aspergillosis	Effective air (HEPA) filters, no plants in the environment

Table 4.
Prevention of pneumonia in the immunosuppressed patients.

measures of pneumonia in the ISP. For example, vaccination practices against influenza virus and Streptococcal disease created an impact on the morbidity and mortality, and perhaps the incidence, of CAP; however, better stimulation of specific immune responses with improved vaccines and more widespread use of these vaccines for the protection of elderly and ISP is needed [40].

4.7 Non-tuberculosis mycobacterial (NTM) infections

Non-tuberculosis mycobacteria (NTM) infections are common in ISP. From approximately 125 environmental saprophytic NTM agents, 20 different pathogenic NTM species have been isolated as pneumonia agents in ISP [41]. The clinical findings in patients with NTM infections are respiratory signs, skin and soft tissue infections, musculoskeletal infections, systemic symptoms, and catheter-related symptoms, while the most common findings are lymphadenitis associated with lung and cutaneous involvement. NTM infections can be easily confused with TB. NTM infections should be considered, and differential diagnoses must be sought for in the case of TB unresponsive to treatment [42, 43]. The clinical and microbiological criteria for diagnosing pulmonary NTM infection, published by ATS/IDSA in 2007, are shown in **Table 5** [44].

Because of difficulties in reporting NTM infections, incidence data in the transplant population are not far from estimates. Limited data show a frequency of 0.16–0.38% in kidney transplant recipients, 0.24–2.8% among heart transplant recipients, and 0.46–8.0% in lung transplant recipients [43, 45]. In a series of 253 patients with a median post-transplant follow-up of 2 years, NTM was isolated from at least one culture in 22%, but only 2.5% needed treatment [43]. Rapidly growing NTM species are reported more frequently, especially in ISP who have undergone abdominal surgery. Likewise, M. avium complex (MAC) infection develops more frequently in individuals with underlying pulmonary disease, such as bronchiectasis [41]. Antimicrobial therapy in NTM infections usually encompasses a multidrug regimen. Dual drug therapy is usually standard; however, when the disease is life-threatening and the bacterial load is high, combination therapy with three agents may be indicated [46].

Specific sub-populations: While fever, cough, and dyspnea were the most frequent symptoms in heart transplant recipients (HTR), *de novo* ventricular dysfunction was

Clinical (both criteria required)
1. High-resolution computed tomography (HRCT) scan showing pulmonary symptoms, such as nodular or cavitary opacities on chest radiograph, or multifocal bronchiectasis with many small nodules (A, I)
and
2. Ruling out alternative diagnoses (A, I)
Microbiological
• Positive culture results from at least two different sputum samples (A, II).
• If sputum cultures are not diagnostic, repeat sputum acid-fast bacillus smears and cultures (C, III),
• or
• Positive cultures from at least one bronchial wash or lavage (C, III),
• or
• Lung biopsy with mycobacterial histopathological features and biopsy showing positive cultures for NTM or mycobacterial histopathological features (granulomatous inflammation or acid-fast bacillus) and one or more sputum culture positive for NTM or bronchial wash (A, II).

Table 5.
Diagnostic criteria of pulmonary non-tuberculosis mycobacterium (NTM) infection published by ATS/IDSA in 2007 [44].

rare [47]. Provided that ISPs are at high risk for infections. Artificial intelligence and machine learning are transforming infection testing and have significant potential to intervene challenging situations observed in ISP [48].

4.8 Radiological characteristics

Chest radiographs may be normal, or mild interstitial reticular streaks may be seen. Images obtained via CXR and CT may reveal nonspecific findings in children. Interpretations of the images of pulmonary infiltrates can suggest agents from bacteria, viruses, and fungi, or non-infectious causes, such as alveolar hemorrhage, pulmonary edema, fluid overload, or malignant processes (**Table 6**) [30].

Relation of causative agents and radiographic characteristics: The flora in the respiratory tract of ISP with chronic obstructive pulmonary disease (COPD), diabetes mellitus (DM), and chronic renal failure (CRF) may change due to frequent hospital admissions. In these patient groups, *H. influenzae*, *S. pneumoniae*, MRSA, *K. pneumoniae,* and *P. aeruginosa* can be isolated in the respiratory tract flora in some cases [49]. A radiographic image of a patient with pneumonia caused by *Acinetobacter* species is shown in **Figure 1**.

Pleural infections and pleurisy due to NTM: NTM pleuritis is a rare presentation. In a systematic review of patients with pleural infections caused by NTM (PINTM) in 41 years (between 1980 and 2021), Bachar et al. reported that PINTM has a predilection for immunocompetent individuals and ISP, with or without chronic lung disease [50]. These infections have a grave outcome and a high risk of complications, requiring surgical interventions besides anti-NTM treatment.

Treatment options for the infection caused by these viruses are limited and largely supportive. The efficacy of antiviral treatments has been demonstrated in patients who are not immunosuppressed. Amantadine and rimantadine can reduce the duration and severity of the disease, when started within the first 48 hours of treatment of influenza. It has also been reported that early initiation of neuraminidase inhibitors

HRCT findings	Clinical problem	Probable causative agents
Lobar infiltration	HIV/AIDS (CD4 > 200 cells/microL) Solid organ transplantation	Semi-invasive aspergillosis *S. aureus*
Ground-glass opacities	HIV/AIDS (CD4 < 200 cells/microL) Hematopoietic stem cell transplantation	Pneumocystis pneumonia CMV
Interstitial infiltration	Neutropenia Hematopoietic stem cell transplantation HIV/AIDS	Invasive pulmonary aspergillosis CMV Pneumocystis pneumonia
Multiple small nodules	Hematopoietic stem cell transplantation HIV/AIDS	CMV Fungi Herpes simplex virus Varicella zoster virus
Halo sign	Neutropenia	Invasive pulmonary aspergillosis
Budding tree	HIV/AIDS Organ transplantation	Bacterial pneumonia Tuberculosis Non-tuberculosis Mycobacteriae
Lymphadenopathies	HIV/AIDS Organ transplantation	Pneumocystis pneumonia Mycobacterium avium-intracellulare complex

Table 6.
Probable causative agents in the immunosuppressed patients in line with high-resolution computed tomography (HRCT) and clinical findings.

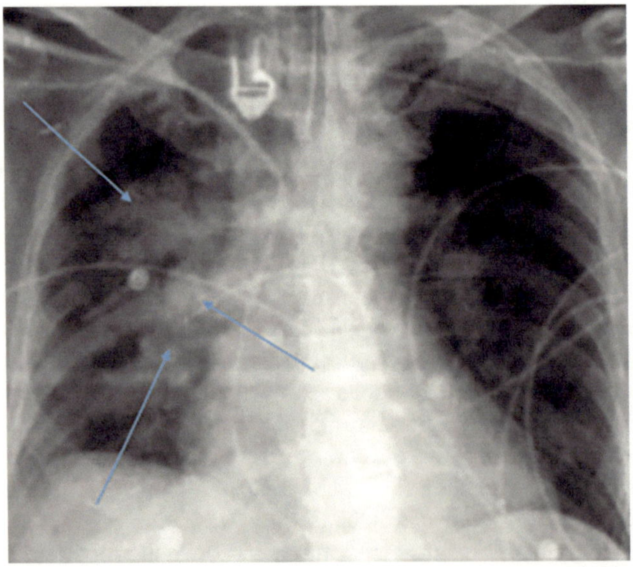

Figure 1.
Chest X-ray of a patient with pneumonia caused by Acinetobacter species (right parahilar consolidation area) (arrows).

(zanamivir and oseltamivir) may be beneficial in influenza A and B infections. Aerosolized ribavirin has also been reported to be effective in RSV and parainfluenza virus infections in published case reports.

4.9 Acute respiratory distress syndrome (ARDS) and infections in ISP

ARDS is a frequent complication of severe viral pneumonia, such as influenza and COVID-19. Like other immunosuppressive conditions, severe viral pneumonia predisposes patients to secondary invasive fungal infections (IFIs). Steroid therapy is commonly used to improve these patients' respiratory distress, but it is also associated with secondary bacterial infections and IFIs [51]. An important example is high incidence of ARDS in severe Legionnaires' disease (LD) [52]. ICU patients with LD necessitate MV and vasopressor use for ARDS and acute kidney injury (AKI) commonly. The prevalence of severe ARDS requiring intubation ranges from 50 to 80%. ARDS and multifocal pneumonia ensue in a majority of patients with severe LD [53].

Patients with COVID-19 who are in need of respiratory support for ARDS have a high risk (>50%) of VAP, mostly due to gram-negative bacteria [54]. Potential factors increasing VAP incidence include immunodeficiency, prolonged ventilation, exposure to immunosuppressants, understaffing, lapses in prevention processes, and overdiagnosis.

4.10 Efficacy of vaccination and ISP

Many conditions triggering immune suppression are associated with different levels of vaccination effectiveness. The response rates to pneumococcal vaccination were assessed in four different treatment groups (mesalamine, azathioprine, infliximab, and infliximab plus azathioprine) in ISP due to inflammatory bowel disease (IBD) [55]. Anti-TNF therapy reduces the response to anti-pneumococcal vaccine in those with IBD. All patients with IBD should therefore be vaccinated before starting anti-TNF therapy. ISP receiving treatment with infliximab or different combinations significantly decreased the likelihood of responding to vaccination.

Clinical and immunological effects of the administration of the bacterial therapeutic polycomponent vaccine Immunovac-VP4 have been assessed for allergen-specific immunotherapy (ASIT) of hay fever [56]. In brief, an 8.5-fold lower incidence of acute respiratory infections was registered in patients receiving combination therapy compared to the control group.

Storek et al. postulated that immunization of the recipient and the donor before transplantation can have a greater effect in enhancing post-transplant antibody immunity than manipulating GVHD, changing conditioning, or increasing the lymphocyte count in the graft [57]. Post-transplant antibody levels are regulated primarily by pre-transplantation levels both in the recipient and the donor.

5. Conclusion

In conclusion, an increasing number of patients are immunosuppressed, and lung infections can often be more complicated in ISP than in other populations throughout the world. This condition, therefore, prompts special attention, experience, and follow-up for the approach in these conditions. It can be difficult to distinguish between infectious and non-infectious agents. Pneumococci and some other organisms are known to colonize the respiratory system in ISP worldwide. In addition to the treatment of lung diseases in ISP, the correct management of the underlying disease is essential. Sound strategies for prevention, coupled with expedient diagnosis and management of these infections, are prerequisites to alleviate the damage to the population as a whole.

Author details

Canan Akman[1], Göksu Afacan Ozturk[2], Feride Sinem Akgun[3], Bilgen Ozkaya[4] and Ozgur Karcıoglu[5]*

1 Department of Emergency Medicine, Canakkale Onsekiz Mart University, Canakkale, Turkey

2 Department of Emergency Medicine, Istanbul Aydin University, Istanbul, Turkey

3 Department of Emergency Medicine, Okan University Faculty of Medicine, Istanbul, Turkey

4 Department of Emergency Medicine, Losante Children's And Adult Hospital, Ankara, Turkey

5 Department of Emergency Medicine, Istanbul Education and Research Hospital, University of Health Sciences, Istanbul, Turkey

*Address all correspondence to: okarcioglu@gmail.com

References

[1] Ramirez JA, File TM Jr. Pulmonary infections in adults: Pulmonary infections in immunocompromised patients. Family Physician Essentials. 2025;**550**:23-29

[2] Marangu D, Zar HJ. Childhood pneumonia in low-and-middle-income countries: An update. Paediatric Respiratory Reviews. 2019;**32**:3-9. DOI: 10.1016/j.prrv.2019.06.001

[3] Brands X, Haak BW, Klarenbeek AM, et al. Concurrent immune suppression and hyperinflammation in patients with community-acquired pneumonia. Frontiers in Immunology. 2020;**11**:796. DOI: 10.3389/fimmu.2020.00796. Erratum in: Front Immunol. 2020;11:626667

[4] Yun KW, Wallihan R, Juergensen A, Mejias A, Ramilo O. Community-acquired pneumonia in children: Myths and facts. American Journal of Perinatology. 2019;**36**(S 02):S54-S57. DOI: 10.1055/s-0039-1691801

[5] American College of Emergency Physicians Clinical Policies Subcommittee (Writing Committee) on Community-Acquired Pneumonia, Smith MD, Fee C, Mace SE, Maughan B, Perkins JC Jr, et al. Clinical policy: Critical issues in the management of adult patients presenting to the emergency department with community-acquired pneumonia. Annals of Emergency Medicine. 2021;**77**(1):e1-e57. DOI: 10.1016/j.annemergmed.2020.10.024

[6] Seymann G, Barger K, Choo S, et al. Clinical judgement versus the pneumonia severity index in making the admission decision. The Journal of Emergency Medicine. 2008;**34**:261-268

[7] Chean D, Windsor C, Lafarge A, et al. Severe community-acquired pneumonia in immunocompromised patients. Seminars in Respiratory and Critical Care Medicine. 2024;**45**(2):255-265. DOI: 10.1055/s-0043-1778137

[8] Facchini L, Martino R, Ferrari A, et al. Degree of mucositis and duration of neutropenia are the major risk factors for early post-transplant febrile neutropenia and severe bacterial infections after reduced-intensity conditioning. European Journal of Haematology. 2012;**88**(1):46-51. DOI: 10.1111/j.1600-0609.2011.01724.x

[9] Pata R, Kristeva J, Kosuru B. Pneumonia in transplant recipients: A comprehensive review of diagnosis and management. Cureus. 2024;**16**(11):e73669. DOI: 10.7759/cureus.73669

[10] Surabhi S, Cuypers F, Hammerschmidt S, Siemens N. The role of NLRP3 inflammasome in pneumococcal infections. Frontiers in Immunology. 2020;**11**:614801. DOI: 10.3389/fimmu.2020.614801

[11] Reynolds D, Kollef M. The epidemiology and pathogenesis and treatment of Pseudomonas aeruginosa infections: An update. Drugs. 2021;**81**(18):2117-2131. DOI: 10.1007/s40265-021-01635-6

[12] Santamarina-Fernández R, Fuentes-Valverde V, Silva-Rodríguez A, García P, Moscoso M, Bou G. *Pseudomonas aeruginosa* vaccine development: Lessons, challenges, and future innovations. International Journal of Molecular Sciences. 2025;**26**(5):2012. DOI: 10.3390/ijms26052012

[13] Driscoll JA, Brody SL, Kollef MH. The epidemiology, pathogenesis and treatment of Pseudomonas aeruginosa infections. Drugs. 2007;**67**(3):351-368. DOI: 10.2165/00003495-200767030-00003

[14] Kang CI et al. Bloodstream infections caused by antibiotic resistant gram-negative bacilli: Risk factors for mortality and impact of inappropriate initial antimicrobial therapy on outcome. Antimicrobial Agents and Chemotherapy. 2005;**49**(2):760-766. DOI: 10.1128/AAC.49.2.760-766.2005

[15] Micek ST, Welch EC, Khan J, et al. Resistance to empiric antimicrobial treatment predicts outcome in severe sepsis associated with gram-negative bacteremia. Journal of Hospital Medicine. 2011;**6**(7):405-410. DOI: 10.1002/jhm.899

[16] Thaden JT, Park LP, Maskarinec SA, Ruffin F, Fowler VG Jr, van Duin D. Results from a 13-year prospective cohort study show increased mortality associated with bloodstream infections caused by Pseudomonas aeruginosa compared to other bacteria. Antimicrobial Agents and Chemotherapy. 2017;**61**(6):e02671-e02616. DOI: 10.1128/AAC.02671-16

[17] Ho J, Hussain S, Sparagano O. Did the COVID-19 pandemic spark a public interest in pet adoption? Frontiers in Veterinary Science. 2021;**8**:444

[18] Gujju VR, Akram B, Shibib DR, McGhee MA, Drevets DA. Bordetella bronchiseptica infections in patients with HIV/AIDS: A case report and review of the literature. Medicine (Baltimore). 2021;**100**(51):e28244. DOI: 10.1097/MD.0000000000028244

[19] Williams BJ, Dehnbostel J, Blackwell TS. *Pseudomonas aeruginosa*: Host defence in lung diseases. Respirology. 2010;**15**(7):1037-1056. DOI: 10.1111/j.1440-1843.2010.01819.x

[20] Parker CM et al. Ventilator-associated pneumonia caused by multidrug-resistant organisms or *Pseudomonas aeruginosa*: Prevalence, incidence, risk factors, and outcomes. Journal of Critical Care. 2008;**23**(1):18-26. DOI: 10.1016/j.jcrc.2008.02.001

[21] Li W, Gao M, Yu J. Rising prevalence and drug resistance of *Corynebacterium striatum* in lower respiratory tract infections. Frontiers in Cellular and Infection Microbiology. 2025;**14**:1526312. DOI: 10.3389/fcimb.2024.1526312

[22] Carvalho RV, Lima F, Santos CSD, Souza MC, Silva RSD, Mattos-Guaraldi AL. Central venous catheter-related infections caused by Corynebacterium amycolatum and other multiresistant non-diphtherial corynebacteria in paediatric oncology patients. The Brazilian Journal of Infectious Diseases. 2018;**22**:347-351. DOI: 10.1016/j.bjid.2018.07.004

[23] Silva-Santana G, Silva CMF, Olivella JGB, Silva IF, Fernandes LMO, Sued-Karam BR, et al. Worldwide survey of Corynebacterium striatum increasingly associated with human invasive infections, nosocomial outbreak, and antimicrobial multidrug-resistance, 1976-2020. Archives of Microbiology. 2021;**203**:1863-1880. DOI: 10.1007/s00203-021-02246-1

[24] Orosz L, Sóki J, Kókai D, Burián K. Corynebacterium striatum-Got Worse by a Pandemic? Pathogens. 14 Jun 2022;**11**(6):685. DOI: 10.3390/pathogens11060685

[25] Gonçalves-de-Albuquerque CF, Silva AR, Burth P, Rocco PR, Castro-Faria MV, Castro-Faria-Neto HC.

Possible mechanisms of Pseudomonas aeruginosa-associated lung disease. International Journal of Medical Microbiology. 2016;**306**(1):20-28. DOI: 10.1016/j.ijmm.2015.11.001

[26] Sadikot RT, Blackwell TS, Christman JW, et al. Pathogen-host interactions in *Pseudomonas aeruginosa* pneumonia. American Journal of Respiratory and Critical Care Medicine. 2005;**171**:1209-1223

[27] Kartchner LB, Gode CJ, Dunn JLM, et al. One-hit wonder: Late after burn injury, granulocytes can clear one bacterial infection but cannot control a subsequent infection. Burns. 2019;**45**(3):627-640. DOI: 10.1016/j.burns.2018.08.019

[28] Gonski K, Cohn R, Widger J, McMullan B. Utility of bronchoscopy in immunocompromised paediatric patients: Systematic review. Paediatric Respiratory Reviews. 2020;**34**:24-34. DOI: 10.1016/j.prrv.2020.02.003

[29] Davidson KR, Ha DM, Schwarz MI, Chan ED. Bronchoalveolar lavage as a diagnostic procedure: A review of known cellular and molecular findings in various lung diseases. Journal of Thoracic Disease. 2020;**12**(9):4991-5019. DOI: 10.21037/jtd-20-651

[30] Kasow KA, King E, Rochester R, et al. Diagnostic yield of bronchoalveolar lavage is low in allogeneic hematopoietic stem cell recipients receiving immunosuppressive therapy or with acute graft-versus-host disease: The St. Jude experience, 1990-2002. Biology of Blood and Marrow Transplantation. 2007;**13**(7):831-837. DOI: 10.1016/j.bbmt.2007.03.008

[31] Amalakuhan B, Echevarria KL, Restrepo MI. Managing community acquired pneumonia in the elderly - The next generation of pharmacotherapy on the horizon. Expert Opinion on Pharmacotherapy. 2017;**18**(11):1039-1048. DOI: 10.1080/14656566.2017.1340937

[32] Debes S, Haug JB, De Blasio BF, Lindstrøm JC, Jonassen CM, Dudman SG. Antibiotic consumption in a cohort of hospitalized adults with viral respiratory tract infection. Antibiotics (Basel). 2023;**12**(4):788. DOI: 10.3390/antibiotics12040788

[33] Bassetti M et al. Systematic review of the impact of appropriate versus inappropriate initial antibiotic therapy on outcomes of patients with severe bacterial infections. International Journal of Antimicrobial Agents. 2020;**56**(6):106184. DOI: 10.1016/j.ijantimicag.2020.106184

[34] Harris PNA, Tambyah PA, Lye DC, et al. Effect of piperacillin-Tazobactam vs Meropenem on 30-day mortality for patients with E coli or Klebsiella pneumoniae bloodstream infection and ceftriaxone resistance: A randomized clinical trial. JAMA. 2018;**320**(10):984-994. DOI: 10.1001/jama.2018.12163. Erratum in: JAMA. 2019;321(23):2370

[35] Bensinger WI, Green DJ, Burwick N, Becker PS. A prospective study of lenalidomide monotherapy for relapse after Allo-SCT for multiple myeloma. Bone Marrow Transplantation. 2014;**49**(4):492-495. DOI: 10.1038/bmt.2013.219

[36] Troeman DP, Postma DF, van Werkhoven CH, Oosterheert JJ. The immunomodulatory effects of statins in community-acquired pneumonia: A systematic review. The Journal of Infection. 2013;**67**(2):93-101. DOI: 10.1016/j.jinf.2013.04.015

[37] Ho C, Lau A, Cimon K, Farrah K, Gardam M. Screening, Isolation,

and Decolonization Strategies for Vancomycin-Resistant Enterococci or Extended Spectrum Beta-Lactamase Producing Organisms: A Systematic Review of the Clinical Evidence and Health Services Impact. Ottawa (ON): Canadian Agency for Drugs and Technologies in Health; 2012

[38] Li J, Li Y, Song N, Chen Y. Risk factors for carbapenem-resistant Klebsiella pneumoniae infection: A meta-analysis. The Journal of Global Antimicrobial Resistance. 2020;**21**:306-313. DOI: 10.1016/j.jgar.2019.09.006

[39] Pérez-Galera S, Bravo-Ferrer JM, Paniagua M, et al. COMBACTE-CARE-EURECA team. Risk factors for infections caused by carbapenem-resistant Enterobacterales: An international matched case-control-control study (EURECA). EClinicalMedicine. 2023;**57**:101871. DOI: 10.1016/j.eclinm.2023.101871

[40] Froneman C, Kelleher P, José RJ. Pneumococcal vaccination in immunocompromised hosts: An update. Vaccines (Basel). 2021;**9**(6):536. DOI: 10.3390/vaccines9060536

[41] Doucette K, Fishman JA. Immunocompromised hosts: Nontuberculous mycobacterial infection in hematopoietic stem cell and solid organ transplant recipients. Clinical Infectious Diseases. 2004;**38**:1428-1439

[42] Brown BA, Wallace RJ Jr. Infections due to nontuberculous mycobacteria other than Mycobacterium avium-intracellulare. In: Mandell GL, Bennett JE, Dolin R, editors. Mandell, Douglas and Bennett's Principles and Practice of Infectious Diseases,7th Ed. Philadelphia PA: Churchill-Livingstone; 2010

[43] Knoll BM, Kappagoda S, Gill RR, et al. Non-tuberculous mycobac-terial infection among lung transplant recipients: A 15-year cohort study. Transplant Infectious Disease. 2012;**14**:452-460

[44] Griffith DE, Aksamit T, Brown-Elliot B, et al. An official ATS/IDSA statement: Diagnosis, treatment, and prevention of nontuberculous mycobacterial diseases. American Journal of Respiratory and Critical Care Medicine. 2007;**175**:367-416

[45] Piersimoni C. Nontuberculous mycobacteria infection in solid organ transplant recipients. European Journal of Clinical Microbiology and Infectious Diseases. 2012;**31**:397-403

[46] Sun HY, Singh N. Opportunistic infection-associated immune reconstitution syndrome in transplant recipients. Clinical Infectious Diseases. 2011;**53**:168-176

[47] Ilonze OJ, Ballut K, Rao RS, Jones MA, Guglin M. SARS-CoV-2 infection in heart transplant recipients: A systematic literature review of clinical outcomes and immunosuppression strategies. Heart Failure Reviews. 2022;**27**(5):1653-1663. DOI: 10.1007/s10741-021-10181-y

[48] Tran NK, Kretsch C, LaValley C, Rashidi HH. Machine learning and artificial intelligence for the diagnosis of infectious diseases in immunocompromised patients. Current Opinion in Infectious Diseases. 2023;**36**(4):235-242. DOI: 10.1097/QCO.0000000000000935

[49] Kotloff R, Ahya V, Crawford S. Pulmonary complications of solid organ and hematopoietic stem cell transplantation. State of art. American Journal of Respiratory and Critical Care Medicine. 2004;**170**:22-48

[50] Bachar K, Shulimzon T, Segel MJ. Nontuberculous mycobacteria infections of the pleura: A systematic review. Respiratory Medicine. 2022;**205**:107036. DOI: 10.1016/j.rmed.2022.107036

[51] Ahmadikia K, Hashemi SJ, Khodavaisy S, et al. The double-edged sword of systemic corticosteroid therapy in viral pneumonia: A case report and comparative review of influenza-associated mucormycosis versus COVID-19 associated mucormycosis. Mycoses. 2021;**64**(8):798-808. DOI: 10.1111/myc.13256

[52] Rello J, Allam C, Ruiz-Spinelli A, Jarraud S. Severe Legionnaires' disease. Annals of Intensive Care. 2024;**14**(1):51. DOI: 10.1186/s13613-024-01252-y

[53] Viasus D, Gaia V, Manzur-Barbur C, Carratala J. Legionnaires' disease: Update on diagnosis and treatment. Infectious Disease and Therapy. 2022;**11**:973-986. DOI: 10.1007/s40121-022-00635-7

[54] Fumagalli J, Panigada M, Klompas M, Berra L. Ventilator-associated pneumonia among SARS-CoV-2 acute respiratory distress syndrome patients. Current Opinion in Critical Care. 2022;**28**(1):74-82. DOI: 10.1097/MCC.0000000000000908

[55] Fiorino G, Peyrin-Biroulet L, Naccarato P, et al. Effects of immunosuppression on immune response to pneumococcal vaccine in inflammatory bowel disease: A prospective study. Inflammatory Bowel Diseases. 2012;**18**(6):1042-1047. DOI: 10.1002/ibd.21800

[56] Poddubikova AM, Kostinov MP. Immunovac-VP4 vaccine used in complex allergen-specific immunotherapy of patients with hay fever. Zhurnal Mikrobiologii, Epidemiologii, i Immunobiologii. Jul-Aug 2010;(4):44-48. Russian

[57] Storek J, Viganego F, Dawson MA, et al. Factors affecting antibody levels after allogeneic hematopoietic cell transplantation. Blood. 2003;**101**(8):3319-3324. DOI: 10.1182/blood-2002-05-1376

Chapter 4

Personalized Corticosteroid Treatment for Patients with Severe COVID-19 Pneumonia under the C-Reactive Protein Levels Control

Ildar Lutfarakhmanov, Ekaterina Soloveitchik, Albert Shakirov and Peter Mironov

Abstract

COVID-19 is often complicated by ARDS and pneumonia with respiratory failure. Corticosteroids are a promising treatment option. OBJECTIVE: To assess the feasibility and safety of personalized corticosteroid prescription to reduce the hyperinflammation in adult patients with comorbid diseases. This dual-center prospective comparative study was conducted in the Clinical Infectious Hospital and Clinical Emergency Hospital (Ufa, Republic of Bashkortostan) from May 2020 to May 2021. Patients received corticosteroids during the first 5 days of hospitalization in accordance with the blood levels of the inflammation biomarker C-reactive protein (personalized administration; n = 30) or as a conventional therapy (n = 28). The patients of personalized group had fewer days of respiratory support as compared with patients in conventional group (9.4 [6.2–15.6] vs. 14.3 [7.1–21.4]; p = 0.003]) and no differences in cumulative outcome (persistent respiratory support or death). Daily levels of the C-reactive protein were significantly lower on 2–4 days of hospitalization in the personalized group compared with the conventional group. In critically ill COVID-19 patients with comorbid diseases, a personalized corticosteroid treatment reduced the frequency of treatment ineffectiveness and the duration of life support.

Keywords: COVID-19, ARDS, pneumonia, comorbid disease, corticosteroids, personalized approach, C-reactive protein

1. Introduction

The novel infectious disease COVID-19 is often complicated by respiratory distress syndrome (ARDS) and pneumonia that need respiratory support in the setting of intensive care unit (ICU) [1–4].

The pathophysiology of COVID-19 is still unclear, but diffuse lung injury is seemingly the result of virus cytotoxicity and systemic inflammatory response syndrome. Theoretically, immunomodulatory drugs, including corticosteroids, may have the effect of reducing lung inflammation in COVID-19 and are being investigated as therapeutic approaches for the treatment of pneumonia [5]. Corticosteroids suppress pulmonary and systemic inflammation, accelerate clinical resolution, reduce the incidence of systemic inflammation-related complications such as ARDS and septic shock, reduce the production of tumor necrosis factor and interleukins, and subsequent recruitment of inflammatory cells into the alveolar space [6, 7]. The efficacy and safety of corticosteroids among critically ill adult patients with viral pneumonia remains largely uncertain due to a lack of evidence from randomized clinical trials and uncertain results from observational studies [8]. The pros and cons of corticosteroids in the treatment of COVID-19 remain controversial [9–20]. At the beginning of the pandemic, there was opposition to the use of corticosteroids for severe pneumonia because they could impair immune defenses and inhibit viral clearance [21]. As a contrary, some meta-analyses have demonstrated the therapeutic efficacy of corticosteroids in COVID-19 [22, 23]. As a result, living WHO guidelines on drugs for COVID-19 suggest not to use systemic corticosteroids for patients with non-severe causes (conditional or weak recommendation), because corticosteroids may increase the risk of 28-day mortality (low certainty) [24]. The Brazilian Guidelines suggest against the routine use corticosteroids for COVID-19 patients' treatment (weak recommendation; Level of Evidence very low) [25]. Contrary, the Australian Taskforce and the European Guideline currently recommend considering using systemic corticosteroids as first line treatment in children and adolescents with acute COVID-19 who are receiving oxygen, including mechanically ventilated (MV) children [26, 27].

When using corticosteroids in critically ill patients with COVID-19 pneumonia, the benefits and risks should be investigated; patients with comorbid diseases should be in cautious, and daily dosage and duration of treatment should be as low (short) as possible [22]. The challenge now is to harness the benefits of corticosteroids and reduce side effects, thereby minimizing mortality and reducing ICU hospitalization time [28, 29]. Although the use of corticosteroids was associated with improved outcomes in pneumonia, their ideal dosage, initiation, and duration of use remain uncertain when used regardless of the individual inflammatory response. The aim of this study was to assess the feasibility and safety of a personalized approach to the prescription of corticosteroids, considering the profile of the inflammation biomarker C-reactive protein (CRP) in reducing the need for respiratory support and the duration of treatment in the ICU in patients with COVID-19 associated pneumonia and comorbid diseases.

2. Materials and methods

This prospective, non-randomized, controlled clinical trial was conducted in accordance with the Declaration of Helsinki (as revised in 2013) in the Infectious Diseases Hospital and the Emergency Hospital (Ufa, Republic of Bashkortostan). The protocol was designed in accordance with the Recommendations for Interventional Trials 2013 statement. Due to the mixed study design, no written informed consent was obtained. An institutional ethics review board of Bashkir State Medical University (Ufa, Republic of Bashkortostan, Russia) approved this study (approval number: № 10/15.12.2021). The flow diagram of the study is shown in **Figure 1**.

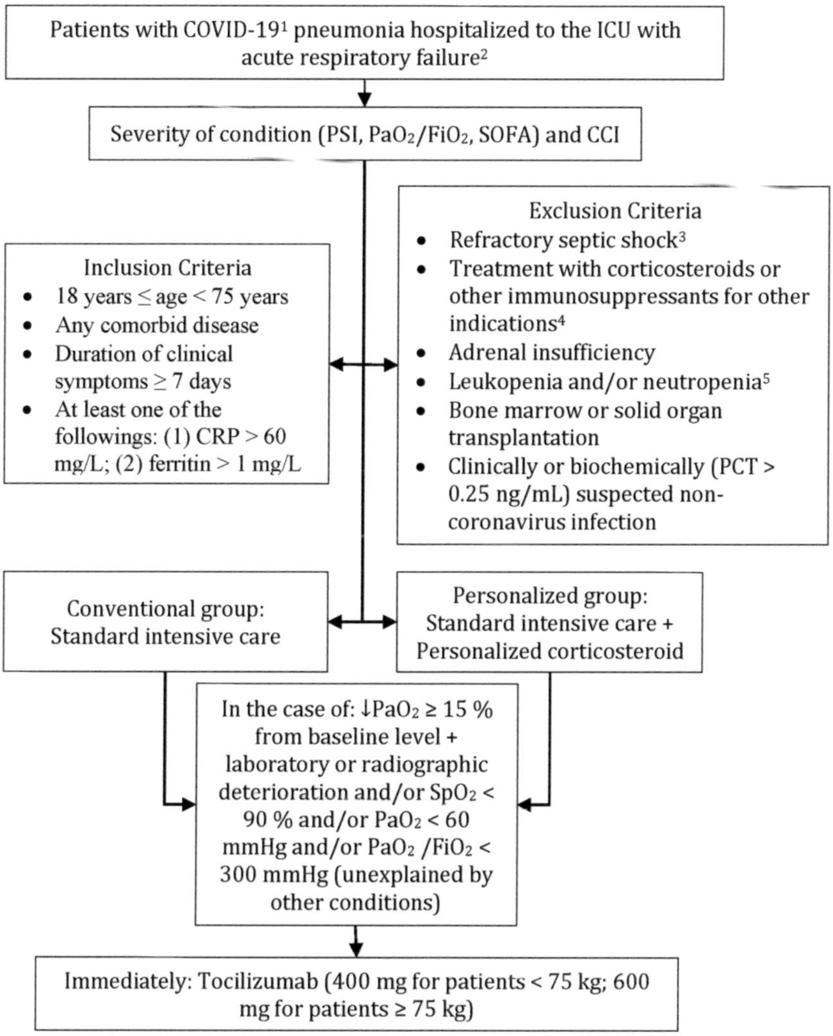

Figure 1.
Flowchart of the study. Note. [1]High suspicion (clinical and radiographic [focal opacity or infiltrate on chest radiograph or CT scan] features, epidemiological history, absence of other infection) or confirmed by a positive polymerase chain reaction (PCR) test in nasal and pharyngeal swabs, or lower respiratory tract aspirate. [2]PaO_2/FiO_2 < 200 mmHg (SpO_2 < 90% when breathing room air or < 95% by inhalation of 2 L of oxygen through nasal cannulas). [3]Need for norepinephrine treatment at doses greater than 0.1 μg/kg/min and/or the use of vasopressor(s) at equivalent doses. The patients with no evidence of circulatory insufficiency at the time of admission whose condition required vasopressor medication after initiation of respiratory support were included provided that: (1) circulatory failure due to exposure to MV and sedatives; (2) blood lactate levels below 4 mmol/L; (3) norepinephrine doses below 0.25 μg/kg/min. [4]Pre-hospitalization use of more than 15 mg/day of prednisolone (or equivalent) for more than 30 days or other immunosuppressive medications. [5]Leukopenia < 1×10^9/L and/or neutropenia <0.5×10^9/L. CCI, Charslon Comorbidity Index; CRP, C-reactive protein; FiO_2, inspired oxygen fraction; ICU, Intensive Care Unit; PaO_2, arterial oxygen pressure; PCR, polymerase chain reaction; PCT, procalcitonin; PSI, Pulmonary Severity Index; SOFA, Sequential Organ Failure Assessment; SpO_2, oxygen blood saturation.

2.1 Corticosteroid administration

Patients with COVID-19 pneumonia and respiratory support received corticosteroids at the dosage and duration of administration according to the daily level of the inflammation biomarker CRP compared to standard intensive care. In the conventional therapy group the use and dosage of corticosteroids were determined by the attending physician on the basis of the interim guidelines of the Ministry of Health of the Russian Federation [30]. In the personalized therapy group the algorithm for dosing, titration and duration of corticosteroids use was selected on the basis of individual CRP levels based on retrospective data [31]. Blood CRP levels were measured during the first 5 days of hospitalization:

- If the CRP level was greater than 200 mg/L, then the patient received 0.3 mg/kg dexamethasone or an equivalent dose of oral prednisolone;
- If the CRP level was between 151 and 200 mg/L, the patient received 0.15 mg/kg dexamethasone or an equivalent dose of prednisolone;
- If the CRP level was between 101 and 150 mg/L, then the patient received 0.1 mg/kg dexamethasone or an equivalent dose of prednisolone;
- If the CRP level was between 50 and 100 mg/L, then the patient received 0.05 mg of dexamethasone or an equivalent dose of prednisolone;
- If the CRP level was less than 50 mg/L, or if the patient's respiratory and general condition improved sufficiently within 4 days of treatment to consider transfer from the ICU, corticosteroids were discontinued. To do this, the following criteria should be presented: spontaneous respiration or low flow oxygen therapy; PaO_2/FiO_2 ratio greater than 200 mmHg; regression of organ failure.

2.2 Outcomes

The primary cumulative outcome included persistent respiratory support or death. Preliminarily defined secondary outcomes included (1) the length of respiratory support measured over a daily basis; (2) episodes of nosocomial infection reported during treatment in the ICU; (3) levels of the inflammation biomarker CRP.

2.3 Statistical analysis

Statistical data processing was performed using the MedCalc software package (v 11.3.1.0, Belgium). Continuous variables are presented as median and 25–75% interquartile range; the categorized variables are represented as absolute values (n) and relative frequency (percentage). Cross-sectional comparisons were made using the Mann-Whitney U-test for nonparametric variables and Pearson's χ^2-test or Fisher's exact test for the corresponding categorized variables. P values less than 0.05 were accepted as statistically significant.

2.4 Patients and settings

From May 2020 to May 2021, a total of 65 adult patients with laboratory-confirmed COVID-19 and/or diagnosed with International Classification of Diseases U07.1, version 10, admitted to the ICU for respiratory support, were consecutively included in this study. Patients who were transferred to another hospital (n = 2) or died (n = 5) in the first 24 hours of hospitalization were excluded from the study,

Variables	Conventional therapy group	Personalized therapy group	p value
Age, years	63 (52–67)	65 (53–73)	0.395
Sex, male/female	15/13	15/15	0.824
BMI, kg/m^2	29 (25–30)	30 (27–32)	0.081
Hypertension	15 (53.6)	14 (46.7)	0.603
Diabetes	5 (17.9)	6 (20.0)	0.840
Obesity	10 (35.7)	11 (36.7)	0.937
Heart Diseases	10 (35.7)	13 (43.3)	0.578
Lung Diseases	3 (10.7)	2 (6.7)	0.665
Kidney Diseases	2 (7.1)	1 (3.3)	0.605
Liver Diseases	1 (3.6)	1 (3.3)	1.000
Oncology	2 (7.1)	2 (6.7)	1.000
CCI >3	10 (35.7)	9 (30.0)	0.647

Note. BMI, body mass index; CCI, Charlson Comorbidity Index.

Table 1.
Demographic variables of patients.

so 28 patients were included in the conventional therapy group and 30 patients in the personalized therapy group. Thirty (51.7%) patients were men, the mean age of the patients was 64 years and the mean body mass index was 29 kg/m^2; arterial hypertension, heart disease, and obesity were the most common comorbid diseases (**Table 1**). PCR test results were positive in 52 (89.6%) patients. There were no significant differences in age, sex, body mass index, and comorbidities between the patient groups.

3. Results

The majority of patients (54; 93.1%) had bilateral pneumonia at the time of admission. Some patients had a PaO_2/FiO_2 index of more than 300 mmHg at the time of hospitalization, but subsequently, the index decreased to less than 200 up to 100 mmHg (**Table 2**).

All patients with acute respiratory failure received respiratory support and all critically ill patients received non-invasive or invasive MV (**Table 3**).

There were no significant differences in the need for respiratory support between the patient groups. Vasopressor treatments were given equally to patients in the personalized or conventional therapy groups. Primary cumulative outcome was observed in 12 (40.0%) patients in the personalized therapy group compared to 17 (60.7%) in the conventional therapy group. The duration of respiratory support was significantly longer in the conventional therapy group. During the ICU treatment, 9 (15.5%) patients had episodes of nosocomial infection, half as long in the personalized therapy group. Daily CRP levels were significantly lower in the personalized therapy group compared with the conventional therapy group on days 2–4 of hospitalization (**Table 4**).

Variables	Conventional therapy group	Personalized therapy group	p value
MBP, mmHg	82 (70–91)	87 (76–94)	0.078
HR, beat/min	85 (70–110)	86 (72–105)	0.834
RR, breath/min	27 (24–31)	26 (21–31)	0.339
Body temperature, °C	37.7 (36.6–39.0)	37.7 (36.9–38.9)	1.000
PaO_2/FiO_2, mmHg	132 (87–230)	139 (90–204)	0.688
Leukocytes, $\times 10^9$/L	8.6 (6.9–10.5)	8.6 (6.6–10.8)	1.000
Lymphocytes, $\times 10^9$/L	0.9 (0.4–1.3)	0.7 (0.7–1.4)	0.063
Platelets, $\times 10^9$/L	208 (161–270)	220 (160–274)	0.440
PCT, ng/mL	0.5 (0.3–0.8)	0.6 (0.4–1.0)	0.175
Glucose, mmol/L	7.7 (6.7–10.2)	8.1 (6.6–10.8)	0.431
Lactate, mmol/L	2.1 (1.9–2.4)	1.9 (1.7–2.7)	0.062
D-dimer, mg/L	1570 (903–3260)	2449 (1101–4468)	0.005
SOFA, score	6.1 (3.0–9.3)	5.5 (3.1–8.3)	0.428

Note. FiO_2, inspired oxygen fraction; HR, heart rate; MBP, mean blood pressure; PaO_2, arterial oxygen pressure; PCT, procalcitonin; RR, respiration rate; SOFA, Sequential Organ Failure Assessment.

Table 2.
Clinical and laboratory variables of patients.

Variables	Conventional therapy group	Personalized therapy group	p value
HFO	3 (10.7)	4 (13.3)	0.070
NIV	12 (42.9)	10 (33.4)	0.325
MV	13 (46.4)	16 (53.3)	0.304
Persistent respiratory support or death	17 (60.7)	12 (40.0)	0.118
Duration of respiratory support, days	14.3 (7.1–21.4)	9.4 (6.2–15.6)	0.003
Nosocomial infection	3 (10.7)	6 (20.0)	0.473

Note. HFO, high-flow oxygen; MV, mechanical ventilation; NIV, non-invasive ventilation.

Table 3.
Treatment modalities and outcomes.

Variables	Conventional therapy group	Personalized therapy group	p value
First day	155 (108–230)	148 (105–205)	0.597
Second day	208 (118–230)	118 (94–169)	0.001
Third day	135 (79–190)	75 (69–115)	0.001
Fourth day	86 (63–141)	59 (54–83)	0.001
Fifth day	87 (61–139)	87 (54–91)	0.989

Table 4.
C-reactive protein levels (mg/L).

4. Discussion

During the pandemic, we have witnessed changes in the standards of care. The proportion of patients with hyperinflammation decreased from 65% in 2020 to 27% in 2022, while the proportion of patients treated with corticosteroids increased from 25% in 2020 up to 70% in 2022. Dexamethasone has previously been shown to exacerbate the body's hyperinflammatory response [32–34]. Low-dose hydrocortisone did not significantly reduce treatment failure, defined as 21-day mortality or persistent respiratory support with high-flow oxygen therapy (HFO) or MV, among critically ill patients with acute respiratory failure associated with COVID-19 [10]. In another study, early use of short-duration, low-to-moderate dosage methylprednisolone was the more accurate immunomodulatory treatment and brought more benefits to severe patients with COVID-19 [20]. Also, the results of the COVIDICUS randomized clinical trial showed that high-dose dexamethasone did not significantly improve 60-day survival among ICU patients with COVID-19-related acute hypoxemic respiratory failure [35]. These findings support current interim clinical guidelines for the treatment of patients with COVID-19 pneumonia with low-dose dexamethasone (6 mg daily for 10 days). Recently published data have confirmed the benefits of using corticosteroids in the treatment of severe forms of COVID-19. The controlled, open-label trial conducted by RECOVERY working group compared high-dose (20 mg daily) versus standard-dose (6 mg daily) of dexamethasone in hospitalized patients with hypoxia. The 28-day mortality rate was higher in the high-dose group than in the standard-dose group (19 vs. 12%) [36]. In the meta-analysis of REACT working group, administration of corticosteroids compared with placebo, resulted in lower mortality of critically ill patients with COVID-19 [37]. In the international multicenter COVID STEROID 2 trial, 12 mg daily dosing of dexamethasone as compared with 6 mg daily dosing did not resulted in significantly different life-support-free days among patients with COVID-19 and severe hypoxemia [38]. In the Bayesian analysis of COVID STEROID 2, the difference for life-support-free days was 1.3 days [39, 40]. The chance of being alive without life support was 64% for those who received 6 mg of dexamethasone, as compared with a 94% chance for those who received 12 mg of dexamethasone. A multicenter, open-label, randomized trial of adult patients with COVID-19-associated ARDS who received high-dose (20 mg/day) or standard-dose (6 mg/d) dexamethasone, showed the absolute difference of life-support-free days of 0.81 days [41]. Despite these results, the benefits or harms of high-dose dexamethasone in patients with COVID-19-associated ARDS are unclear.

The body's response to COVID-19 can be pro- or anti-inflammatory [42, 43]. In the absence of a standard definition of hyperinflammation, some biomarkers have shown abnormalities consistent with this state [44–47]. In particular, patients with hyperinflammation had the highest levels of CRP, a standard biomarker of inflammation associated with COVID-19. The hyperinflammatory pattern of ARDS was confirmed by elevated interleukin-6 levels [48]. In our study, we hypothesized that increased corticosteroid use was associated with a decrease in the prevalence of hyperinflammation, and we assessed this association in 30 patients who personified dexamethasone use in the first 5 days of treatment and compared with 28 control patients who received conventional therapy. In our study, we confirmed the presence of a hyperinflammatory pattern in pneumonia. Using CRP levels, we found that hyperinflammation had an increased incidence of respiratory failure, requiring HFO up to MV.

The empirical use of corticosteroids in severe ARDS remains controversial, and the results of clinical trials vary considerably. A multicenter, randomized controlled trial showed that patients with moderate-to-severe ARDS treated with dexamethasone had more life-supporting-free days and lower mortality [49]. Different subphenotypes within ARDS showed different responses to corticosteroid treatment. The hyperinflammatory phenotype showed a higher mortality rate, and a retrospective analysis of ARDS in COVID-19 observed the heterogeneity of treatment effect to corticosteroids, with improved mortality in the hyperinflammatory phenotype and worse mortality in the hypoinflammatory phenotype [15]. Although the empirical use of corticosteroids remains controversial in all patients with severe ARDS, there are likely distinct subgroups of ARDS in whom it is clinically effective.

The results of our clinical trial suggest that the personalized approach to the prescribing, dosing, and duration of corticosteroids under the control of the inflammation biomarker CRP is effective and safe in the treatment of severe COVID-19 associated pneumonia requiring ICU hospitalization and respiratory support in terms of reducing the incidence of cumulative outcome, defined as persistent respiratory support and/or death among critically ill patients with comorbid diseases. The personalized approach provided a more precise strategy for drug therapy in comparison with universal temporary guidelines. A limitation of the study was the difficulty to assess the effect of other treatments administered concomitantly with corticosteroids. However, the patients with COVID-19 who did not receive corticosteroids experienced longer hospital stays [11]. Given the hard period of pandemic in which the study was conducted, some data were incomplete or missing.

5. Conclusion

In our cohort of critically ill patients with COVID-19-associated pneumonia and comorbid diseases, the personalized approach to corticosteroid administration was associated with no significant reduction in the incidence of treatment failure (defined as persistent respiratory support and/or death) from 60.7 to 40.0%. Using the commonly available inflammation biomarker C-reactive protein, we found that hyperinflammation was associated with a high risk of respiratory failure and required a significantly longer duration of respiratory support (14.3 versus 9.4 days).

Author details

Ildar Lutfarakhmanov*, Ekaterina Soloveitchik, Albert Shakirov and Peter Mironov
Bashkir State Medical University, Ufa, Russia

*Address all correspondence to: lutfarakhmanov@yandex.ru

References

[1] Grasselli G, Zangrillo A, Zanella A, COVID-19 Lombardy ICU Network. Baseline characteristics and outcomes of 1591 patients infected with SARS-CoV-2 admitted to ICUs of the Lombardy Region, Italy. Journal of the American Medical Association. 2020;**323**(16):1574-1581. DOI: 10.1001/jama.2020.5394

[2] Wu Z, McGoogan JM. Characteristics of and important lessons from the coronavirus disease 2019 (COVID-19) outbreak in China: Summary of a report of 72 314 cases from the Chinese Center for Disease Control and Prevention. Journal of the American Medical Association. 2020;**323**(13):1239-1242. DOI: 10.1001/jama.2020.2648

[3] Yang X, Yu Y, Xu J, et al. Clinical course and outcomes of critically ill patients with SARS-CoV-2 pneumonia in Wuhan, China: A single-centered, retrospective, observational study. Lancet Respiratory Medicine. 2020;**8**(5):475-481. DOI: 10.1016/S2213-2600(20)30079-5

[4] Wu C, Chen X, Cai Y, et al. Risk factors associated with acute respiratory distress syndrome and death in patients with coronavirus disease 2019 pneumonia in Wuhan, China. Journal of the American Medical Association Internal Medicine. 2020;**180**(7):934-943. DOI: 10.1001/jamainternmed.2020.0994

[5] Sanders JM, Monogue ML, Jodlowski TZ, et al. Pharmacologic treatments for coronavirus disease 2019 (COVID-19): A review. Journal of the American Medical Association. 2020;**323**(18):1824-1836. DOI: 10.1001/jama.2020.6019

[6] De Pascale G, Bello G, Antonelli M. Steroids in severe pneumonia: A literature review. Minerva Anestesiologica. 2011;**77**(9):902-910

[7] Annane D, Sébille V, Troché G, et al. A 3-level prognostic classification in septic shock based on cortisol levels and cortisol response to corticotropin. Journal of the American Medical Association. 2000;**283**(8):1038-1045. DOI: 10.1001/jama.283.8.1038

[8] Arabi YM, Fowler R, Hayden FG. Critical care management of adults with community-acquired severe respiratory viral infection. Intensive Care Medicine. 2020;**46**(2):315-328. DOI: 10.1007/s00134-020-05943-5

[9] Angus DC, Derde L, Al-Beidh F, et al. Effect of hydrocortisone on mortality and organ support in patients with severe COVID-19: The REMAP-CAP COVID-19 corticosteroid domain randomized clinical trial. Journal of the American Medical Association. 2020;**324**(13):1317-1329. DOI: 10.1001/jama.2020.17022

[10] Dequin PF, Heming N, Meziani F, CAPE COVID Trial Group and the CRICS-TriGGERSep Network. Effect of hydrocortisone on 21-day mortality or respiratory support among critically ill patients with COVID-19: A randomized clinical trial. Journal of the American Medical Association. 2020;**324**(13):1298-1306. DOI: 10.1001/jama.2020

[11] Fadel R, Morrison AR, Vahia A, Henry Ford COVID-19 Management Task Force. Early short-course corticosteroids in hospitalized patients with COVID-19. Clinical Infectious Disease. 2020;**71**(16):2114-2120. DOI: 10.1093/cid/ciaa601

[12] CMP J, MEL F, FFA V, Metcovid Team. Methylprednisolone as adjunctive

therapy for patients hospitalized with coronavirus disease 2019 (COVID-19; Metcovid): A randomized, double-blind, phase IIb, placebo-controlled trial. Clinical Infectious Disease. 2021;**72**(9):e373-e381. DOI: 10.1093/cid/ciaa1177

[13] Lu X, Chen T, Wang Y, et al. Adjuvant corticosteroid therapy for critically ill patients with COVID-19. Critical Care. 2020;**24**(1):241. DOI: 10.1186/s13054-020-02964-w

[14] Laikitmongkhon J, Tassaneyasin T, Sutherasan Y, et al. A comparative study between methylprednisolone versus dexamethasone as an initial anti-inflammatory treatment of moderate COVID-19 pneumonia: An open-label randomized controlled trial. BMC Pulmonary Medicine. 2024;**24**(1):562. DOI: 10.1186/s12890-024-03364-4

[15] Issak ER, Amin MM. Timing of corticosteroids in non-severe non-hospitalized COVID-19 patients: Open-label, two-center, randomized controlled study (TICS-COV19 study). Korean Journal of Internal Medicine. 2023;**38**(2):207-217. DOI: 10.3904/kjim.2022.232

[16] Taher A, Lashkari M, Keramat F, et al. Comparison of the efficacy of equivalent doses of dexamethasone, methylprednisolone, and hydrocortisone for treatment of COVID-19-related acute respiratory distress syndrome: A prospective three-arm randomized clinical trial. Wiener Medizinische Wochenschrift. 2023;**173**(5-6):140-151. DOI: 10.1007/s10354-022-00993-4

[17] Salvarani C, Massari M, Costantini M, et al. Intravenous methylprednisolone pulses in hospitalised patients with severe COVID-19 pneumonia: A double-blind, randomised, placebo-controlled trial. European Respiratory Journal. 2022;**60**(4):2200025. DOI: 10.1183/13993003.00025-2022

[18] Granholm A, Kjær MN, Munch MW, et al. Long-term outcomes of dexamethasone 12 mg versus 6 mg in patients with COVID-19 and severe hypoxaemia. Intensive Care Medicine. 2022;**48**(5):580-589. DOI: 10.1007/s00134-022-06677-2

[19] Toroghi N, Abbasian L, Nourian A, et al. Comparing efficacy and safety of different doses of dexamethasone in the treatment of COVID-19: A three-arm randomized clinical trial. Pharmacological Reports. 2022;**74**(1):229-240. DOI: 10.1007/s43440-021-00341-0

[20] Yang L, Peng L, Wu W, et al. Low-to-moderate dosage and short term use of corticosteroids benefit patients with severe COVID-19 infections. Frontiers of Microbiology. 2022;**13**:953328. DOI: 10.3389/fmicb.2022.953328

[21] Russell CD, Millar JE, Baillie JK. Clinical evidence does not support corticosteroid treatment for 2019-nCoV lung injury. Lancet. 2020;**395**(10223):473-475. DOI: 10.1016/S0140-6736(20)30317-2

[22] van Paassen J, Vos JS, Hoekstra EM, et al. Corticosteroid use in COVID-19 patients: A systematic review and meta-analysis on clinical outcomes. Critical Care. 2020;**24**(1):696. DOI: 10.1186/s13054-020-03400-9

[23] Zayed Y, Barbarawi M, Ismail E, et al. Use of glucocorticoids in patients with acute respiratory distress syndrome: A meta-analysis and trial sequential analysis. Journal of Intensive Care. 2020;**8**:43. DOI: 10.1186/s40560-020-00464-1

[24] Agarwal A, Hunt B, Stegemann M, et al. A living WHO guideline on drugs for COVID-19. BMJ. 2020;**370**:m3379. DOI: 10.1136/bmj.m3379

[25] Falavigna M, Colpani V, Stein C, et al. Guidelines for the pharmacological treatment of COVID-19. The task-force/consensus guideline of the Brazilian Association of Intensive Care Medicine, the Brazilian Society of Infectious Diseases and the Brazilian Society of Pulmonology and Tisiology. Revista Brasileira de Terapia Intensiva. 2020;**32**(2):166-196. DOI: 10.5935/0103-507x.20200039

[26] Fraile Navarro D, Tendal B, Tingay D, et al. Clinical care of children and adolescents with COVID-19: Recommendations from the national COVID-19 clinical evidence taskforce. Medical Journal of Australia. 2022;**216**(5):255-263. DOI: 10.5694/mja2.51305

[27] Chalmers JD, Crichton ML, Goeminne PC, et al. Management of hospitalised adults with coronavirus disease 2019 (COVID-19): A European Respiratory Society living guideline. European Respiratory Journal. 2021;**57**(4):2100048. DOI: 10.1183/13993003.00048-2021

[28] Shang L, Zhao J, Hu Y, et al. On the use of corticosteroids for 2019-nCoV pneumonia. Lancet. 2020;**395**(10225):683-684. DOI: 10.1016/S0140-6736(20)30361-5

[29] Vecchié A, Batticciotto A, Tangianu F, et al. High-dose dexamethasone treatment for COVID-19 severe acute respiratory distress syndrome: A retrospective study. Internal and Emergency Medicine. 2021;**16**(7):1913-1919. DOI: 10.1007/s11739-021-02800-1

[30] Temporary Guidelines. Prevention, Diagnosis and Treatment of New Coronavirus Infection (COVID-19). Version 3. Ministry of Health of the Russian Federation; 2020. Времснные_MP_COVID-19_03.03.2020_(версия_3)_6-6.pdf (in Russ)

[31] Torres A, Sibila O, Ferrer M, et al. Effect of corticosteroids on treatment failure among hospitalized patients with severe community-acquired pneumonia and high inflammatory response: A randomized clinical trial. Journal of the American Medical Association. 2015;**313**(7):677-686. DOI: 10.1001/jama.2015.88

[32] Longobardo A, Snow TAC, Montanari C, et al. COVID-19 and non COVID ARDS patients demonstrate a distinct response to low dose steroids - A retrospective observational study. Journal of Critical Care. 2021;**62**:46-48. DOI: 10.1016/j.jcrc.2020.11.012

[33] Chen H, Xie J, Su N, et al. Corticosteroid therapy is associated with improved outcome in critically ill patients with COVID-19 with hyperinflammatory phenotype. Chest. 2021;**159**(5):1793-1802. DOI: 10.1016/j.chest.2020.11.050

[34] Ho KS, Narasimhan B, Difabrizio L, et al. Impact of corticosteroids in hospitalised COVID-19 patients. BMJ Open Respiratory Research. 2021;**8**(1):e000766. DOI: 10.1136/bmjresp-2020-000766

[35] Bouadma L, Mekontso-Dessap A, Burdet C, COVIDICUS Study Group. High-dose dexamethasone and oxygen support strategies in intensive care unit patients with severe COVID-19 acute hypoxemic respiratory failure: The COVIDICUS randomized clinical trial. JAMA Internal Medicine. 2022;**182**(9):906-916. DOI: 10.1001/jamainternmed.2022.2168

[36] RECOVERY Collaborative Group. Higher dose corticosteroids in patients admitted to hospital with COVID-19 who are hypoxic but not requiring ventilatory support (RECOVERY): A randomised, controlled, open-label, platform trial. Lancet. 2023;**401**(10387):1499-1507. DOI: 10.1016/S0140-6736(23)00510-X

[37] WHO Rapid Evidence Appraisal for COVID-19 Therapies (REACT) Working Group, JAC S, Murthy S, Diaz JV, et al. Association between Administration of Systemic Corticosteroids and Mortality among Critically ill patients with COVID-19: A meta-analysis. JAMA. 2020;**324**(13):1330-1341. DOI: 10.1001/jama.2020.17023

[38] Munch MW, Myatra SN, Vijayaraghavan BKT, COVID STEROID 2 Trial Group. Effect of 12 mg vs 6 mg of dexamethasone on the number of days alive without life support in adults with COVID-19 and severe hypoxemia: The COVID STEROID 2 randomized trial. Journal of the American Medical Association. 2021;**326**(18):1807-1817. DOI: 10.1001/jama.2021.18295

[39] Granholm A, Munch MW, Myatra SN, et al. Dexamethasone 12 mg versus 6 mg for patients with COVID-19 and severe hypoxaemia: A pre-planned, secondary Bayesian analysis of the COVID STEROID 2 trial. Intensive Care Medicine. 2022;**48**(1):45-55. DOI: 10.1007/s00134-021-06573-1

[40] Granholm A, Munch MW, Andersen-Ranberg N, et al. Heterogeneous treatment effects of dexamethasone 12 mg versus 6 mg in patients with COVID-19 and severe hypoxaemia – Post hoc exploratory analyses of the COVID STEROID 2 trial. Acta Anaesthesiologica Scandinavica. 2023;**67**(2):195-205. DOI: 10.1111/aas.14167

[41] Maláska J, Stašek J, Máca J, et al. Effects of two different dexamethasone dosing regimens on ventilator-free days and long-term mortality in COVID-19 patients with moderate-to-severe ARDS: The REMED randomized clinical trial. European Journal of Medical Research. 2024;**29**(1):616. DOI: 10.1186/s40001-024-02215-6

[42] Remy KE, Brakenridge SC, Francois B, et al. Immunotherapies for COVID-19: Lessons learned from sepsis. Lancet Respiratory Medicine. 2020;**8**(10):946-949. DOI: 10.1016/S2213-2600(20)30217-4

[43] Notz Q, Schmalzing M, Wedekink F, et al. Pro- and anti inflammatory responses in severe COVID-19-induced acute respiratory distress syndrome-an observational pilot study. Frontiers in Immunology. 2020;**11**:581338. DOI: 10.3389/fimmu.2020.581338

[44] Caricchio R, Gallucci M, Dass C, Temple University COVID-19 Research Group. Preliminary predictive criteria for COVID-19 cytokine storm. Annals of the Rheumatic Disease. 2021;**80**(1):88-95. DOI: 10.1136/annrheumdis-2020-218323

[45] Manson JJ, Crooks C, Naja M, et al. COVID-19-associated hyper inflammation and escalation of patient care: A retrospective longitudinal cohort study. The Lancet Rheumatology. 2020;**2**(10):e594-e602. DOI: 10.1016/S2665-9913(20)30275-7

[46] Reddy K, Rogers AJ, McAuley DF. Delving beneath the surface of hyperinflammation in COVID-19. The Lancet Rheumatology. 2020;**2**(10):e578-e579. DOI: 10.1016/S2665-9913(20)30304-0

[47] Zeng F, Huang Y, Guo Y, et al. Association of inflammatory markers

with the severity of COVID-19: A meta-analysis. International Journal of Infectious Diseases. 2020;**96**:467-474. DOI: 10.1016/j. ijid.2020.05.055

[48] Sinha P, Furfaro D, Cummings MJ, et al. Latent class analysis reveals COVID-19-related acute respiratory distress syndrome subgroups with differential responses to corticosteroids. American Journal of Respiratory Critical Care Medicine. 2021;**204**(11):1274-1285. DOI: 10.1164/rccm.202105-1302OC

[49] Villar J, Ferrando C, Martínez D, et al. Dexamethasone treatment for the acute respiratory distress syndrome: A multicentre, randomised controlled trial. The Lancet Respiratory Medicine. 2020;**8**(3):267-276. DOI: 10.1016/S2213-2600(19)30417-5

Chapter 5

Vascular Graft Infections

Haris Vukas, Samra Kadić-Vukas, Sumeja Ćatić, Ruvejda Dizdarević, Farah Dedović, Hana Muslić, Melica Imamović-Bošnjak, Dragan Piljić and Haris Vranić

Abstract

Treatment of AAA and RAAA remains demanding in terms of technical performance, intraoperative, early, and late postoperative complications. Colicured intramural thrombi are usually found, which in RAAA disintegrate into the retroperitoneum. EVAR and TEVAR procedures are also not free from a suitable infectious medium. Are the early signs of air around the graft only postprocedural, or are they the first signs of an inflammatory response and possible Postoperative laboratory inflammatory findings, MRI and CTA, as well as the patient's physical condition, suggest a higher infectious risk after elective and emergency surgery. How to diagnostically monitor and treat patients after R(T)AAA and immunocompromised patients after elective (T)AAA? graft infection.

Keywords: vascular, infection, chronic, graft, AAA

1. Introduction

Vascular graft infections (VGIs) are a serious and often difficult-to-manage complication in vascular surgery, carrying high risks for patient morbidity and mortality. As the use of both synthetic and biological graft materials has become routine in procedures such as bypass surgery for peripheral arterial disease, aortic aneurysm repair, and coronary artery disease, the potential for infection has become a growing concern in clinical practice. Although VGIs are relatively rare, their consequences can be severe, including graft failure, sepsis, limb loss, and prolonged hospitalization. The pathophysiology of these infections involves complex interactions between microbial pathogens and the surface of the implanted graft material, often resulting in biofilm formation and resistance to both host immune defenses and antibiotic therapy [1]. Despite progress in surgical techniques and antimicrobial treatment, VGIs remain a major risk factor for poor clinical outcomes, and management often requires a combination of long-term antibiotics, surgical debridement, or even complete graft removal. One of the ongoing challenges in clinical settings is that VGIs can present with subtle or nonspecific symptoms, and the lack of standardized diagnostic criteria can delay timely recognition and appropriate treatment. Furthermore, there is still no universally accepted treatment algorithm, which leads to variation in clinical management between institutions. This chapter aims to provide an in-depth overview of VGIs by discussing their pathogenesis, risk factors, clinical presentation, diagnostic strategies, and therapeutic options, drawing on both current research and real-world clinical experience to help guide prevention and improve patient outcomes. Vascular graft and endograft infections (VGEIs) are typically multifactorial, shaped by a complex interplay of patient-related, surgical, and environmental factors, which complicates the estimation of their true incidence—a topic that will be addressed in detail in subsequent sections, including incidence by graft type and anatomical location [2].

2. Pathogenesis of vascular graft infections

Bacterial infections are still the main cause of vascular graft infections, while fungi like *Candida albicans* and *Aspergillus*, along with *mycoplasma* and *mycobacteria*, are less common. Over the years, however, the types of infections we see have started to change. In older studies, *Staphylococcus aureus* was responsible for about half of all vascular graft infections, but that number has gone down, and now *Staphylococcus epidermidis* is behind roughly 60% of these cases [3]. Vascular graft infections are generally classified as either early or late. Most of them happen within the first 4 months after surgery, which we refer to as early infections [4]. During this time, the most common culprits are coagulase-positive *Staphylococcus aureus* and Gram-negative bacteria like Escherichia coli, Proteus, and *Pseudomonas aeruginosa*. On the other hand, infections that show up more than 4 months after surgery are called late infections, which are usually caused by coagulase-negative *Staphylococcus epidermidis*. Fungal infections can also occur, but they are much less common [5]. *Staphylococcus aureus* is known for being highly virulent, mainly because it produces enzymes that cause hemolysis and tissue damage. It makes coagulase, along with several toxic proteolytic enzymes that break down proteins. Another important feature is its ability to produce a mucin layer, an extracellular glycoprotein that helps it stick to prosthetic grafts. This mucin also acts as a protective barrier, shielding the bacteria from antibiotics and the immune system's phagocytic cells. On the other hand, *Staphylococcus epidermidis*, which normally lives harmlessly on the skin, is much less aggressive. It does not produce coagulase, has limited ability to invade tissues, and generally only causes problems when there is a foreign material like a prosthetic graft present, which it can use as a surface to grow on [6]. Early vascular graft infections (VGEIs) usually happen because of contamination during surgery or because bacteria were already present in the aneurysmal thrombus at the time of implantation. On the other hand, late VGEIs are more often caused by bacteria spreading through the bloodstream, usually from infections in the urinary or respiratory tract or from bacterial translocation or contamination during procedures like catheterization.

When it comes to aorto-enteric (AEnF), aorto-esophageal (AEsF), and aorto-bronchial fistulas (ABF), the exact causes are not fully understood. However, several factors have been suggested, such as reduced blood flow to the walls of nearby organs due to blocked arteries, or the constant pressure and erosion caused by an aneurysm or pseudoaneurysm, especially if there is an ongoing endoleak. These fistulas might also result from direct trauma during surgery, poor tunneling of the graft, erosion from repeated contact, or penetration caused by a graft that is too large [7]. The quality of material incorporation, which depends on tissue ingrowth and healing, also plays a critical role. This may explain why VEGI might occur more frequently than VG infections (VGI), as the endograft fabric lacks tissue ingrowth and is surrounded only by thrombotic material, unlike vascular grafts [7, 8].

3. Risk factors

Patients most at risk for graft infections are usually older and often have other serious health problems—like diabetes, kidney failure (uraemia), liver issues such as jaundice, or obesity. People taking steroids or those with weakened immune systems are also more vulnerable. One of the biggest warning signs is if there is already a wound or skin infection near the surgical site, since that can easily lead to infection of the graft itself. The risk of prosthetic vascular graft infection is strongly linked to superficial and wound infections [8]. Certain complications after surgery—like fluid buildup (seromas or lymphoceles) or bleeding that forms a hematoma—can also raise the risk of infection [8]. This is especially true when the graft is placed in the groin area. That part of the body is close to the perineum, has skin folds, and tends to collect fluid or blood after procedures like femoral arteriography, all of which can increase the chance of bacteria getting in. Waiting a bit longer between groin procedures and the actual surgery may help lower the risk [9]. To prevent infection, it is important to use careful surgical technique and give antibiotics around the time of surgery [9]. If a graft does become infected, acting quickly is essential. Treatment usually involves removing the infected graft and, when possible, using the patient's own tissue to rebuild the blood vessel. With the right approach, many patients recover fully and stay free of infection over the long term [9].

The incidence of graft infection is higher in emergency surgeries, particularly those performed for ruptured abdominal aortic aneurysms or acutely ischemic limbs. Additionally, early reoperation, including wound and graft exploration, has been shown to significantly elevate graft infection rates and should be avoided whenever possible. Extra caution is necessary in these cases to minimize the risk of infection.

4. Diagnosis

4.1 Clinical features

The way infections present in patients can vary widely, depending on how severe the infection is and how the patient's immune system responds. Some patients might only have vague, nonspecific symptoms like fever, tiredness, or bacteremia, while others develop much more serious and potentially life-threatening complications, such as bleeding problems or septic shock. Local signs of infection, like redness, swelling, or pus, can sometimes help point to a diagnosis, but these signs are not always there [10]. Because of that, diagnosing infections often means relying on symptoms that are not clearly linked to any one cause, which can make things more difficult. This is especially challenging when a patient does not show the usual signs of infection, requiring clinicians to stay alert and consider infection even when it is not obvious. On top of this, the process is often made harder by the fact that there is no widely agreed-upon approach to diagnosing and managing these infections. As some researchers have pointed out, this leads to big differences in how patients are treated from one hospital to another [11]. Surgical site infections (SSIs) are a well-known risk, and they can affect both the surface and deeper tissues of a wound. But just because a wound looks fine does not mean everything is okay; an infection can still be present, which is why a full clinical assessment is so important. The problem is, early signs of infection often look a lot like normal inflammation that happens after surgery. That makes it even more important for doctors to make careful, informed judgments.

All of this points to the need for clearer, evidence-based guidelines that help clinicians make more consistent decisions. New diagnostic tools like specific biomarkers, better imaging technologies, and molecular tests are starting to close that gap, offering hope for faster and more accurate diagnoses.

4.2 Ultrasound (US)

The most popular, affordable, non-invasive imaging technique for detecting VGEI-related abnormalities is US. Pseudoaneurysm, sustained gas presence (if present after >7 weeks), and purely anechoic fluid collections (if present after >3 months after surgery) are US characteristics of VGEI [12]. It can distinguish between abscess formation and hemorrhage, which makes it a good primary imaging screening modality, especially for superficial peripheral VG. However, a VGEI cannot be ruled out due to the lack of periprosthetic collections in the US. Additionally, US can guide puncture for bacteriological purposes and allow for the investigation of graft thrombosis, which may be the initial indication of VGEI [13]. Nevertheless, US has a significant interoperator variability and a limited predictive value.

4.3 Computed tomography angiography (CTA)

Since CTA can visualize the characteristic features of VGEI, it has long been the standard imaging method for diagnosing VGEI [14]. Intravenous contrast, when used with images obtained in the arterial phase, may reveal certain signs like ectopic gas, fluid, soft tissue enhancement, pseudoaneurysm, focal bowel thickening, and discontinuation of the aneurysmal wall. 36 Additionally, in the arterial phase, it may be possible to detect contrast passage from the aorta to the digestive tract in cases of AEnF.

4.4 Magnetic resonance angiography (MRA)

For the diagnosis of VGEI, MRA has not been studied as thoroughly as CTA; however, a number of studies have indicated that MRA provides better anatomical and functional information than CTA, including tissue characterization. Acquiring 18F-FDG-PET simultaneously or sequentially with MRA offers additional quantitative molecular functional information about the inflammatory lesion, precise localization, and anatomical changes with motion correction. A VGEI is strongly suggested by collections with a hypo-intense signal in T1 and a hyperintense signal in T2 after six postoperative weeks [15].

4.5 Diagnostic criteria

To address the limitations of existing classifications, the Management of Aortic Graft Infection (MAGIC) group has developed a framework consisting of major and minor criteria based on clinical, surgical, radiological, and laboratory findings. When vascular graft and endograft infection (VGEI) is suspected, a thorough assessment of the patient's clinical condition, signs of infection, and comorbidities in accordance with the MAGIC criteria is advised (**Table 1**).

According to the established diagnostic criteria, a suspicion of vascular graft or endograft infection (VGEI) arises when either one major criterion or two minor criteria from three different categories are present. A definitive diagnosis requires at least one major criterion combined with at least one additional criterion from a different category.

Criteria	Clinical/surgical	Radiology	Laboratory
Major	Open wound with exposed graft or communicating sinus	Perigraft fluid on CT scan $\geq$3 months after insertion	Organisms recovered from an explanted graft
	Open wound with exposed graft or communicating sinus	Perigraft gas on CT scan $\geq$7 weeks after insertion	Organisms recovered from an intraoperative specimen
	Fistula development, e.g., aorto-enteric or aorto-bronchial	Increase in perigraft gas volume demonstrated on serial imaging	Organisms recovered from a percutaneous, radiologically guided aspirate of perigraft fluid
	Graft insertion in an infected site, e.g., fistula, mycotic aneurysm, or infected pseudoaneurysm		
Minor	Localized clinical features of graft infection, e.g., erythema, warmth, swelling, purulent discharge, pain	Suspicious perigraft gas/fluid soft tissue inflammation; aneurysm expansion; pseudoaneurysm formation; focal bowel wall thickening; discitis/osteomyelitis; suspicious metabolic activity on FDG PET/CT; radiolabeled leukocyte uptake	Blood culture(s) positive and no apparent source except graft infection
	Fever $\geq$38°C with graft infection as the most likely cause		Abnormally elevated inflammatory markers, e.g., erythrocyte sedimentation rate, C-reactive protein, white cell count

Table 1.
The MAGIC classification.

For example, while a fever of $\geq$38°C is frequently observed in affected patients, it is not specific to VGEI and must be interpreted cautiously—especially when other possible causes of fever have not been excluded. Similarly, sepsis or systemic inflammatory response syndrome (SIRS) may result from non-infectious or unrelated infectious processes and typically reflects a combination of clinical, laboratory, and hemodynamic changes. Symptoms like anorexia, lethargy, and general malaise can also be seen in patients with aortic graft or endograft infections, but on their own, they are nonspecific and insufficient for diagnosis. These challenges underscore the importance of integrating clinical findings with imaging, microbiological, and laboratory data to establish a reliable diagnosis of VGEI.

Intraoperative fluids surrounding a graft may resemble pus due to their yellowish or cloudy appearance, but this can also occur for non-infectious reasons, with negative microbiological cultures. The presence of pus cells confirmed via direct microscopy qualifies as a major criterion. Additionally, direct communication between non-sterile sites and the prosthesis—such as an aorto-enteric fistula (AEnF), aorto-bronchial fistula (ABF), implantation of a stent graft in an already infected field (e.g., an infected aneurysm), or exposed grafts in deep open wounds—indicates graft infection [2].

5. Therapeutical strategies

Centralizing the care of patients with vascular graft or endograft infections (VGEI) is clearly essential, given the rarity of the condition, the complexity of its diagnosis and treatment, and the potentially severe clinical outcomes. Referral to specialized, high-volume centers with demonstrated experience in managing VGEI is strongly recommended. These centers should have access to a multidisciplinary team, including specialists in vascular and cardiovascular surgery, radiology, angiology, infectious diseases, and microbiology. A coordinated, team-based approach is critical to ensure accurate diagnosis, timely surgical intervention, appropriate antimicrobial therapy, and optimal long-term outcomes.

5.1 Antimicrobial therapy

An essential component of treating VGEI is antimicrobial therapy. To treat infection and sepsis during the acute phase, aggressive antimicrobial therapy with a wide range of antibiotics or medicines targeted against the most likely infecting organisms is recommended. The possibility of a biofilm covering the graft material and the local epidemiology of resistance patterns must be taken into account when selecting an antibiotic treatment. Antifungal medications should be added in some circumstances, particularly when visceral fistulas are present. If at all feasible, the spectrum should be reduced after the relevant infecting organisms are identified [16].

The optimal duration of antimicrobial therapy for vascular graft or endograft infections (VGEI) remains a matter of debate. In cases where the prosthetic material can be completely removed and thorough debridement of all infected tissue is possible, a minimum of 2 weeks of intravenous antibiotics, followed by an oral regimen for an additional 2–4 weeks, is generally recommended. However, when the infected graft is replaced with a new vascular graft, a more prolonged course of antimicrobial therapy, typically 4–6 weeks, is advised to prevent recurrence [17]. In some situations, especially when the infection is complex or caused by low-virulence pathogens, treatment durations of 3–6 months have been proposed. In rare cases, up to 1 year of therapy may be considered. For patients who are not suitable surgical candidates due to significant comorbidities, lifelong suppressive antibiotic therapy may be necessary [18]. This approach can also be considered for patients with low-grade infections caused by less aggressive organisms, particularly if the infection is responsive to antimicrobial therapy and there are no complicating factors.

While complete eradication of infection may not always be achievable, long-term or even lifelong antimicrobial therapy can offer acceptable disease control and improve quality of life in selected patients.

Since carriage is prolonged, especially in patients receiving antibiotics, patients with multidrug-resistant (MDR) bacteria (like MRSA, but not methicillin-resistant coagulase-negative staphylococci, extended-spectrum beta-lactamase-producing Enterobacteriaceae, or glycopeptide-resistant enterococci) should be isolated and kept isolated throughout their hospital stay. Although it is not unique to MDR bacteria, gloves must be used when handling any biological material (gown for any touch with the patient, mask for pulmonary colonization or infection). To lessen the chance of the bacterium spreading to other patients, both colonized and infected patients should be treated in the same room.

5.2 Surgical treatment

In the past, the gold standard for preventing recurrent infection was complete removal of the diseased VG or EG, debridement and washing of the affected region with an antiseptic solution, and extra-anatomic repair (EAR) outside the contaminated field. If at all feasible, this process should be carried out in two steps. This strategy, however, raises the possibility of issues like stump blowout and is not always practical or simple. As a result, the majority of writers now favor an in situ reconstruction (ISR) using material that is resistant to infection in conjunction with vigorous artery bed debridement, targeted antimicrobial treatment, and removal of the infected graft material [19]. The outcomes of ISR are typically at least as good as those of extra-anatomic repair.

The timing of surgery is closely tied to the patient's clinical condition. For hemodynamically unstable patients experiencing acute bleeding or septic shock, an endovascular "bridging to surgery" approach can be considered to manage aorto-bronchial or aorto-esophageal fistulas. While current clinical guidelines for vascular graft infections do not specify the optimal timing for surgery, recommendations from guidelines for left-sided infective endocarditis might offer adaptable insights [20].

Historically, the standard treatment involved extra-anatomical bypass combined with extensive debridement and complete removal of the infected graft. However, the invasiveness of this procedure has led to high perioperative mortality rates, prompting the development of alternative approaches for infection control. One such alternative includes selective debridement combined with irrigation techniques.

Given the lack of a universal solution, surgeons must refine their expertise in debridement and adopt the most appropriate strategy tailored to each patient's needs.

6. Complications

Vascular graft infections (VGIs) present significant challenges in both diagnosis and management. The complications arising from these infections are dependent on several factors, including the location of the graft, the type of infection, and the overall health status of the patient. While the majority of vascular graft infections are manageable with appropriate intervention, they can lead to serious, life-threatening outcomes if not promptly addressed. This section delves into the specific complications associated with various types of vascular graft infections, particularly those involving the aorta, femoral arteries, and upper extremity vasculature.

6.1 Aortic graft infections and associated complications

Aortic graft infections are among the most critical, given the vital role of the aorta in systemic circulation and the high-pressure blood flow within it. Infections in this region often lead to catastrophic complications if left untreated. One of the most concerning outcomes is the formation of aorto-enteric fistulas (AEF), a direct communication between the aorta and the gastrointestinal tract. AEF often begins with a small "herald" bleed and can quickly progress to massive, fatal hemorrhage. Early diagnosis with CT angiography is critical, and initial bleeding control with endovascular techniques like TEVAR or stent balloon tamponade can be lifesaving [21].

Another life-threatening complication specific to aortic graft infections is the development of aorto-esophageal fistulas. These fistulas form when the infected graft erodes through the esophagus, creating an abnormal connection between the two structures. Additionally, esophageal fistulas can also occur in patients with aortic graft infections. Early diagnosis is crucial, especially in patients with prior TEVAR procedures. These fistulas are characterized by the formation of an abnormal connection between the graft and the esophagus, leading to chronic low-grade fever, dysphagia, aspiration pneumonia, and malnutrition. While these symptoms may develop more insidiously than the more acute aorto-esophageal fistulas, esophageal fistulas are associated with significant long-term morbidity due to the difficulty in managing the infection and restoring normal gastrointestinal function. Any such patient with GI bleeding or sepsis should prompt urgent evaluation. Temporary control with TEVAR may be needed, but definitive open surgery is essential [22, 23].

Aortic graft infections can cause serious problems beyond fistulas. In situ reconstruction (ISR) had fewer reinfections and better survival than extra-anatomical reconstruction (EAR) or conservative treatment, making ISR the preferred option. Using the patient's own veins did not show better outcomes than synthetic grafts. Infected grafts may form pseudoaneurysms and bulges that can rupture and cause life-threatening bleeding [24].

Septic embolization is a serious complication, where infected material or clot fragments are carried through the bloodstream, potentially causing distant abscesses, ischemic organ damage, or infarctions. Finally, the spread of infection can lead to septic shock, where the systemic inflammatory response to the infection leads to hemodynamic collapse and multiple organ dysfunction [24].

6.2 Femoral artery graft infections and associated complications

Femoral artery graft infections are often associated with peripheral artery disease or trauma repair, and while they tend to present with more localized symptoms, the complications can still be severe. Local infection can progress to the formation of abscesses, which may require surgical drainage and prolonged antibiotic therapy. If the infection is not adequately controlled, it may spread to surrounding tissues, including the skin and soft tissues, resulting in cellulitis and further tissue necrosis.

A particularly dangerous complication of femoral graft infections is the formation of pseudoaneurysms at the graft site, where the infection causes weakening and dilation of the graft, ultimately leading to the risk of rupture. This can result in life-threatening hemorrhage, especially in patients with compromised vascular integrity. Patients with deep groin infections after femoral bypass surgery often have serious health issues like diabetes and heart disease. They found that aggressive wound cleaning combined with early flap coverage helped save more grafts and limbs than older approaches [24, 25].

Additionally, untreated infections can lead to critical limb ischemia (CLI), a condition where blood flow to the affected limb is severely restricted, often necessitating amputation if the infection leads to irreversible tissue damage [25].

Femoral artery graft infections also carry the risk of septic arthritis, particularly when the infection spreads to the adjacent hip joint. This can lead to rapid joint destruction, requiring joint replacement surgery or resulting in permanent disability. Moreover, in cases of persistent infection, the formation of chronic draining sinuses can complicate wound healing, leading to ongoing purulent discharge and delayed recovery [26].

6.3 Upper extremity graft infections and associated complications

Infections of grafts placed in the axillary and brachial arteries are less common but can still present unique challenges due to the anatomical location and functional demands of the upper extremities. One of the most serious complications is neurovascular compression caused by the swelling and abscess formation associated with infection. The brachial and axillary regions contain vital structures, such as the brachial plexus and major blood vessels, and compression can lead to neuropathy or motor dysfunction. This can severely impair limb function, affecting a patient's quality of life [27].

In addition to neurovascular issues, fistula formation is a concern. Infection can lead to the development of an abnormal connection between the graft and surrounding tissues, including veins, which can cause chronic infection or thrombosis. If not treated promptly, this can further compromise vascular access and lead to long-term complications such as chronic venous insufficiency or the need for additional interventions [28].

Another significant risk of upper extremity graft infections is thrombosis within the graft, which may lead to embolization. The infected thrombus can break off and travel distally, causing ischemia in the fingers or hand, and potentially resulting in digital gangrene or amputation. Moreover, in patients who require the graft for dialysis access, the infection can lead to the loss of dialysis access, necessitating the use of alternative access sites and increasing the complexity of the patient's care.

6.4 Lower extremity graft infections and associated complications

Infections of grafts placed in the lower extremities, particularly in patients with peripheral vascular disease or following bypass surgeries, present a unique set of complications. These infections can lead to severe outcomes due to the critical nature of the blood flow in the legs and the need for proper healing to avoid amputations.

Infection-related thrombosis is one of the most significant complications in lower extremity graft infections. As the infection progresses, thrombosis can form within the graft, leading to ischemia and necrosis of the tissue supplied by the affected vessel. This condition is particularly dangerous as it can result in permanent damage to the leg, and in severe cases, necessitate amputation to save the patient's life. The presence of pseudoaneurysms can further complicate the situation, as these can rupture, leading to severe bleeding and hemodynamic instability. Infected grafts that fail to heal may also result in chronic wound infections and non-healing ulcers, which are difficult to manage and often require extended antibiotic therapy and multiple surgical interventions [29].

Septic embolism is another complication that can arise in lower extremity graft infections. Infected material or clot fragments can break off and embolize to distant parts of the body, potentially causing end-organ damage or infarctions. Systemic infection can lead to septic shock, which is associated with high mortality, especially when complicated by multiple organ failure. Limb loss is one of the most devastating complications, particularly when the graft infection causes irreversible tissue damage or when revascularization options are unavailable [30].

Infection of the graft site can also lead to chronic lymphatic complications, including lymphorrhea, where lymphatic fluid leaks from the wound, further complicating the healing process and prolonging recovery. In some cases, lymphedema may develop if the lymphatic channels are compromised during infection or surgery.

7. Perioperative strategies for prevention

A meta-analysis [31] found no evidence that preoperative bathing or showering with antiseptic agents offers any benefit over regular, unmedicated bathing. However, several other measures have been shown to significantly reduce the risk of surgical site infections (SSIs) by up to 51% in patients undergoing open or endovascular elective surgery or elective lower limb amputation. These include maintaining normal body temperature during the perioperative period (normothermia), removing hair the day before surgery, and strictly following aseptic practices in the operating room [31]. Broad-spectrum systemic antibiotics have been shown to significantly lower the risk of wound infections and early graft infections in arterial reconstruction procedures. As a result, perioperative systemic antimicrobial prophylaxis is recommended for all patients undergoing open or endovascular abdominal aortic aneurysm repair. However, extending this prophylaxis beyond 24 hours does not appear to provide any additional benefit [32]. For vascular surgeries, antibiotic prophylaxis should target the bacteria most commonly responsible for SSIs. It is essential to ensure that the antibiotic reaches effective levels in the tissue at the time of incision and remains effective throughout the procedure, to prevent bacterial colonization of damaged tissue or implanted materials. First- or second-generation cephalosporins are most often used because of their good safety profile and their effectiveness against methicillin-susceptible *Staphylococcus aureus, coagulase-negative staphylococci, streptococci*, and certain Gram-negative bacilli. In settings with a high rate of MRSA or coagulase-negative staphylococcal infections, additional antibiotic coverage might be considered. However, studies have not shown a significant reduction in SSI rates when comparing cefazolin combined with vancomycin or daptomycin to cefazolin alone [33]. Antibiotic prophylaxis is most effective when administered before the surgical incision, ideally within 30 minutes. For longer procedures, re-dosing should be performed based on the half-life of the antibiotic used, such as 2 hours for cefuroxime and 4 hours for cefazolin.

8. Conclusion

Vascular graft infections are still one of the most difficult complications in vascular surgery, despite all the progress made in recent years. They not only put patients at serious risk but also place a heavy burden on healthcare systems. While we have seen improvements in surgical techniques, graft materials, and postoperative care, these infections continue to pose major challenges that often require the involvement of multiple specialties. Making an early and accurate diagnosis is essential, but it can be tricky, especially when imaging findings are unclear or cultures come back negative. Using newer diagnostic methods like molecular testing and biomarkers might help us catch these infections sooner and more reliably. Preventing infections in the first place is obviously the best approach, and that still depends on careful surgical technique, clean working conditions, and the right use of antibiotics. At the same time, newer ideas like grafts with antimicrobial coatings or drug-releasing surfaces are promising ways to reduce the chances of bacteria sticking to the graft in the first place. Once an infection is established, though, the treatment can be very complicated. It often means long-term antibiotics and more surgery—sometimes even removing or replacing the graft—which comes with serious risks and stresses for the patient. That is why we need more research into better, less invasive treatment options, and even into tissue-engineered solutions that might change how we approach this problem altogether. If we want to improve outcomes for patients, we have to keep thinking in terms of the whole picture—prevention, diagnosis, and treatment—and we need to keep working together across different disciplines to get there.

Author details

Haris Vukas[1,2]*, Samra Kadić-Vukas[3], Sumeja Ćatić[4], Ruvejda Dizdarević[2], Farah Dedović[2], Hana Muslić[5], Melica Imamović-Bošnjak[3], Dragan Piljić[6] and Haris Vranić[7]

1 Clinic of Cardiovascular Surgery, Clinical Center University of Sarajevo, Sarajevo, Bosnia and Herzegovina

2 Sarajevo School of Science of Technology Medical School, Sarajevo, Bosnia and Herzegovina

3 Cantonal Hospital Zenica, Zenica, Bosnia and Herzegovina

4 Health Center Zenica, Zenica, Bosnia and Herzegovina

5 Medical Faculty, University Zenica, Zenica, Bosnia and Herzegovina

6 Clinic of Cardiovascular Surgery, University Clinical Center Tuzla, Bosnia and Herzegovina

7 Department of Vascular Surgery, General Hospital Sarajevo, Sarajevo, Bosnia and Herzegovina

*Address all correspondence to: haris.vks77@gmail.com

References

[1] Lyons OT, Baguneid M, Barwick TD, et al. Diagnosis of aortic graft infection: A case definition by the Management of Aortic Graft Infection Collaboration (MAGIC). European Journal of Vascular and Endovascular Surgery. 2016;**52**(6):758-763. DOI: 10.1016/j.ejvs.2016.09.007

[2] Chakfé N, Diener H, Lejay A, et al. Editor's choice - European Society for Vascular Surgery (ESVS) 2020 clinical practice guidelines on the Management of Vascular Graft and Endograft Infections [published correction appears in Eur J Vasc Endovasc Surg. 2020;60(6):958. Doi: 10.1016/j.ejvs.2020.07.080]. European Journal of Vascular and Endovascular Surgery. 2020;**59**(3):339-384. DOI: 10.1016/j.ejvs.2019.10.016

[3] Motte S, Bellens B, Rickaert F, Serruys E, Thys JP, Dereume JP. Vascular graft infection caused by aspergillus species: Case report and review of the literature. Journal of Vascular Surgery. 1993;**17**(3):607-612

[4] Kikta MJ, Goodson SF, Bishara RA, Meyer JP, Schuler JJ, Flanigan DP. Mortality and limb loss with infected infrainguinal bypass grafts. Journal of Vascular Surgery. 1987;**5**(4):566-571. DOI: 10.1067/mva.1987.avs0050566

[5] Bandyk DF, Berni GA, Thiele BL, Towne JB. Aortofemoral graft infection due to Staphylococcus epidermidis. Archives of Surgery. 1984;**119**(1):102-108. DOI: 10.1001/archsurg.1984.01390130084015

[6] Geary KJ, Tomkiewicz ZM, Harrison HN, et al. Differential effects of a gram-negative and a gram-positive infection on autogenous and prosthetic grafts. Journal of Vascular Surgery. 1990;**11**(2):339-347. DOI: 10.1067/mva.1990.17626

[7] Kakkos SK, Bicknell CD, Tsolakis IA, Bergqvist D. Editor's choice – Management of secondary aorto-enteric and other abdominal arterio-enteric fistulas: A review and pooled data analysis. European Journal of Vascular and Endovascular Surgery. 2016;**52**(5):770-786. DOI: 10.1016/j.ejvs.2016.08.002

[8] Samson RH, Veith FJ, Janko GS, Gupta SK, Scher LA. A modified classification and approach to the management of infections involving peripheral arterial prosthetic grafts. Journal of Vascular Surgery. 1988;**8**(2):147-153

[9] Goldstone J. The infected infra-renal aortic graft. Acta Chirurgica Scandinavica. Supplementum. 1987;**538**:72-86

[10] Teebken OE, Bisdas T, Assadian O, Ricco JB. Recommendations for reporting treatment of aortic graft infections. European Journal of Vascular and Endovascular Surgery. 2012;**43**(2):174-181. DOI: 10.1016/j.ejvs.2011.11.003

[11] Van Hemelrijck M, Sromicki J, Husmann L, Rancic Z, Hasse B, Carrel TP. Vascular graft infections. Vessel Plus. 2022;**6**:47. DOI: 10.20517/2574-1209.2022.18

[12] Orton DF, LeVeen RF, Saigh JA, et al. Aortic prosthetic graft infections: Radiologic manifestations and implications for management. Radiographics. 2000;**20**(4):977-993. DOI: 10.1148/radiographics.20.4.g00jl12977

[13] Spartera C, Morettini G, Petrassi C, et al. Role of magnetic resonance imaging in the evaluation of aortic graft healing, perigraft fluid collection, and graft infection. European Journal of Vascular Surgery. 1990;**4**(1):69-73. DOI: 10.1016/s0950-821x(05)80041-6

[14] Bruggink JL, Glaudemans AW, Saleem BR, et al. Accuracy of FDG-PET-CT in the diagnostic work-up of vascular prosthetic graft infection. European Journal of Vascular and Endovascular Surgery. 2010;**40**(3):348-354. DOI: 10.1016/j.ejvs.2010.05.016

[15] Shahidi S, Eskil A, Lundof E, Klaerke A, Jensen BS. Detection of abdominal aortic graft infection: Comparison of magnetic resonance imaging and indium-labeled white blood cell scanning. Annals of Vascular Surgery. 2007;**21**(5):586-592. DOI: 10.1016/j.avsg.2007.03.018

[16] Darouiche RO. Treatment of infections associated with surgical implants. The New England Journal of Medicine. 2004;**350**(14):1422-1429. DOI: 10.1056/NEJMra035415

[17] Kahlberg A, Melissano G, Mascia D, Loschi D, Grandi A, Chiesa R. How to best treat infectious complications of open and endovascular thoracic aortic repairs. Seminars in Vascular Surgery. 2017;**30**(2-3):95-102. DOI: 10.1053/j.semvascsurg.2017.11.002

[18] Spiliotopoulos K, Preventza O, Green SY, et al. Open descending thoracic or thoracoabdominal aortic approaches for complications of endovascular aortic procedures: 19-year experience. The Journal of Thoracic and Cardiovascular Surgery. 2018;**155**(1):10-18. DOI: 10.1016/j.jtcvs.2017.08.023

[19] Revest M, Camou F, Senneville E, et al. Medical treatment of prosthetic vascular graft infections: Review of the literature and proposals of a working group. International Journal of Antimicrobial Agents. 2015;**46**(3):254-265. DOI: 10.1016/j.ijantimicag.2015.04.014

[20] Tacconelli E, Cataldo MA, Dancer SJ, et al. ESCMID guidelines for the management of the infection control measures to reduce transmission of multidrug-resistant gram-negative bacteria in hospitalized patients. Clinical Microbiology and Infection. 2014;**20**(Suppl. 1):1-55. DOI: 10.1111/1469-0691.12427

[21] Wong AC, Chou YM, Goh ZNL, Chang KF, Seak CJ. Case report: Aortoesophageal fistula-an extremely rare but life-threatening cardiovascular cause of hematemesis. Frontiers in Cardiovascular Medicine. 2023;**10**:1123305. Published 2023 Apr 20. DOI: 10.3389/fcvm.2023.1123305

[22] Uno K, Koike T, Takahashi S, Komazawa D, Shimosegawa T. Management of aorto-esophageal fistula secondary after thoracic endovascular aortic repair: A review of literature. Clinical Journal of Gastroenterology. 2017;**10**(5):393-402. DOI: 10.1007/s12328-017-0762-z

[23] Jin S, Wei G, Qu X, Li W. Surgical treatment of graft infection combined with aortoesophageal fistula after TEVAR: A retrospective single-center, single-arm study. Journal of Cardiothoracic Surgery. 2024;**19**(1):535. Published 2024 Sep 20. DOI: 10.1186/s13019-024-03109-8

[24] Ge J, Weng C, Zhao J, Yuan D, Huang B, Wang T. Management and clinical outcome of aortic graft infections: A single-center retrospective study. Journal of Clinical Medicine. 2022;**11**(21):6588. Published 2022 Nov 7. DOI: 10.3390/jcm11216588

[25] Herrera FA, Kohanzadeh S, Nasseri Y, Kansal N, Owens EL, Bodor R. Management of vascular graft infections with soft tissue flap coverage: Improving limb salvage rates--a veterans affairs experience. The American Surgeon. 2009;**75**(10):877-881. DOI: 10.1177/000313480907501003

[26] McCready RA, Bryant MA, Divelbiss J, Wack MF, Mattison HR. Chronic femoropopliteal prosthetic graft infection with exposed graft: A case report and review of management. Vascular and Endovascular Surgery. 2009;**43**(5):414-416. DOI: 10.1177/1538574408326265

[27] Lejay A, Koncar I, Diener H, Vega de Ceniga M, Chakfé N. Post-operative infection of prosthetic materials or stents involving the supra-aortic trunks: A comprehensive review. European Journal of Vascular and Endovascular Surgery. 2018;**56**(6):885-900. DOI: 10.1016/j.ejvs.2018.07.016

[28] Tayebi P, Kazemzadeh G, Modaghegh MHS, Kamyar MM, Ravari H. Brachio-basilic upper arm transposition fistulas vs. prosthetic brachio-axillary vascular access grafts-which one is preferred for hemodialysis? Hemodialysis International. 2020;**24**(2):182-187. DOI: 10.1111/hdi.12817

[29] Nguyen LL, Lipsitz SR, Bandyk DF, et al. Resource utilization in the treatment of critical limb ischemia: The effect of tissue loss, comorbidities, and graft-related events. Journal of Vascular Surgery. 2006;**44**(5):971-976. DOI: 10.1016/j.jvs.2006.07.035

[30] Balzer K, Schönebeck I. Odeme nach gefässchirurgischen Eingriffen und deren Therapie [Edema after vascular surgery interventions and its therapy]. Zeitschrift für Lymphologie. 1993;**17**(2):41-47

[31] Stewart AH, Eyers PS, Earnshaw JJ. Prevention of infection in peripheral arterial reconstruction: A systematic review and meta-analysis. Journal of Vascular Surgery. 2007;**46**(1):148-155. DOI: 10.1016/j.jvs.2007.02.065)

[32] Wanhainen A, Verzini F, Herzeele V I, et al. Editor's choice - European Society for Vascular Surgery (ESVS) 2019 clinical practice guidelines on the Management of Abdominal Aorto-iliac Artery Aneurysms [published correction appears in Eur J Vasc Endovasc Surg. 2020;59(3):494. DOI: 10.1016/j.ejvs.2019.11.026.]. European Journal of Vascular and Endovascular Surgery. 2019;**57**(1):8-93. DOI: 10.1016/j.ejvs.2018.09.020

[33] Stone PA, AbuRahma AF, Campbell JR, et al. Prospective randomized double-blinded trial comparing 2 anti-MRSA agents with supplemental coverage of cefazolin before lower extremity revascularization. Annals of Surgery. 2015;**262**(3):495-501. DOI: 10.1097/SLA.0000000000001433), 10.1097/SLA.0000000000001433)

Chapter 6

Diagnosis and Management of Acute Periprosthetic Joint Infections

Taner Karlidag and Omer Halit Keskin

Abstract

Periprosthetic joint infection (PJI) is among the most severe complications associated with total joint arthroplasty (TJA), leading to heightened risks of mortality and morbidity, as well as a diminished quality of life for affected individuals. Early and precise diagnosis of PJI is essential to enable effective treatment and improve outcomes. However, identifying PJI remains a formidable challenge due to the lack of a diagnostic test with absolute reliability. This difficulty is particularly pronounced in cases of acute PJI occurring shortly after surgery, where widespread postoperative inflammation and edema complicate the diagnostic process. Currently, the diagnostic framework for PJI involves integrating multiple sources of information, including clinical evaluation, preoperative serological tests, analysis of aspirated joint fluid, and microbiological and histopathological examination of tissues or fluids obtained intraoperatively. Despite these available methods, there is ongoing debate in the medical community regarding standardized diagnostic protocols. Given these complexities, a multidisciplinary approach is essential to ensure comprehensive management of patients with PJI. Collaborative efforts among orthopedic surgeons, infectious disease specialists, microbiologists, and pathologists are critical to achieving accurate diagnosis and effective treatment planning.

Keywords: acute periprosthetic joint infection, diagnosis, management, multidisciplinary approach, diagnostic tools

1. Introduction

Periprosthetic joint infection (PJI) represents one of the most severe complications following total joint arthroplasty (TJA), significantly contributing to increased mortality [1], morbidity [2], and diminished quality of life [3]. The reported incidence of PJI ranges between 1 and 2% for primary arthroplasty procedures, with rates of 0.97% for total hip arthroplasty (THA) and 1.03% for total knee arthroplasty (TKA) [4, 5]. Notably, PJI is the leading cause of revision surgery for failed total knee arthroplasty, accounting for 16.8–25.2% of cases [6] and ranks as the third most common reason for revision total hip arthroplasty (14.8%) [7]. In addition, using the most recent data, the combined annual hospital costs related to PJI of the hip and knee were estimated to be $1.85 billion by 2030. This includes $753.4 million for THA PJI and $1.1 billion for TKA PJI in that year [8]. Furthermore, there is a projected four-fold increase in the number of TJAs expected by 2030 [9], and with the anticipated four-fold increase in TJA procedures by 2030, the prevalence of PJI is likely to rise substantially [5].

Timely and accurate diagnosis of PJI is crucial for achieving effective treatment and improving patient outcomes [10, 11]. However, the diagnostic process remains challenging due to the absence of a definitive test with perfect accuracy. Diagnosing acute PJI during the early postoperative period is particularly problematic because of the presence of extensive inflammation and edema that may obscure clinical indicators. A delayed or missed diagnosis of PJI can result in the rapid formation of biofilm on the prosthetic implant surface, a process that depends on the specific microorganisms involved.

Biofilm formation on implant surfaces significantly reduces the penetration efficacy of antibiotics and increases microbial resistance, posing a substantial challenge to infection management. Successful treatment strategies must target the eradication of microorganisms residing within the biofilm. Two principal surgical approaches are available to address infection following arthroplasty: (1) removal of the prosthesis to facilitate complete biofilm elimination or (2) aggressive debridement of infected tissue combined with the use of biofilm-active antibiotics, allowing prosthesis retention.

This chapter explores the current approaches and challenges in diagnosing and managing acute PJI, with an emphasis on strategies to optimize outcomes in this complex and evolving field.

2. Definition of acute PJI

The classification of PJIs has evolved over time to identify the timing of infection, the likely causative pathogen, and the most appropriate therapeutic approach. Acute PJI, as outlined in the widely recognized Tsukayama classification [12], is defined as an infection occurring within 4 weeks of the primary arthroplasty or as an acute presentation of symptoms within 4 weeks in a previously well-functioning joint, indicative of hematogenous spread. This temporal definition provides a framework for distinguishing acute infections from other types of PJI and informs the selection of treatment strategies.

3. Diagnosis

Diagnosing PJI presents a persistent and significant challenge for the orthopedic community. The absence of a single, highly reliable diagnostic tool has made it difficult to establish a universally accepted "gold standard" for PJI diagnosis. At present, the diagnostic process relies on a multifaceted approach that integrates clinical evaluation, serological testing, microbiological cultures, histopathological analysis, and advanced molecular diagnostic techniques.

Despite these tools, confirming the presence of infection and accurately identifying the causative organism remains a complex and critical task. An accurate etiological diagnosis is essential to guide targeted therapeutic interventions and optimize patient outcomes. The complexity of PJI diagnosis underscores the importance of a comprehensive diagnostic framework that combines traditional and emerging methods to address this intricate clinical problem effectively.

4. Diagnostic criteria

Currently, there is no universally accepted reference standard for diagnosing PJI. A review of the literature highlights significant variability in diagnostic accuracy, with false-positive culture results from preoperative hip aspirations reported in 3–16% of cases [13]. Similarly, false-positive and false-negative culture rates from tissue biopsies of TKA or THA specimens have been reported at approximately 6 and 10%, respectively [14]. Furthermore, negative intraoperative culture results are observed in 10–30% of suspected cases, complicating the diagnostic process. These limitations have led many surgeons to reconsider the reliability of preoperative joint aspiration and tissue biopsy cultures as definitive diagnostic tools for PJI [15].

The current diagnostic framework for PJI involves a multifaceted approach, combining clinical evaluation, preoperative serological markers, joint aspiration results, and microbiological and histopathological analysis of tissue or fluid samples collected during surgery [16]. However, there remains no consensus on the optimal combination of preoperative and intraoperative tests to definitively confirm or exclude PJI.

In recent years, efforts to develop standardized definitions and diagnostic protocols have gained traction. Notably, the Musculoskeletal Infection Society (MSIS) and the Infectious Diseases Society of America (IDSA) have introduced criteria aimed at standardizing the diagnosis of PJI [17, 18]. These efforts were further refined during a consensus meeting in 2013, where the MSIS definition of PJI was endorsed with slight modifications [19]. More recently, Parvizi et al. proposed an evidence-based diagnostic model with sensitivity and specificity rates of 97.7 and 99.5%, respectively [20].

The criteria outlined by Parvizi et al. [20], classify two positive cultures or the presence of a sinus tract as major diagnostic indicators of PJI. A weighted scoring system was developed based on preoperative and intraoperative findings. Key components include:

- Serological markers:
- Elevated serum C-reactive protein (CRP) >1 mg/dL (2 points)
- D-dimer >860 ng/mL (2 points)
- Erythrocyte sedimentation rate (ESR) >30 mm/h (1 point)
- Synovial fluid analysis:
- White blood cell count (WBC) >3000 cells/mL (3 points)
- Alpha-defensin (AD) (signal-to-cutoff ratio > 1) (3 points)
- Leukocyte esterase (++ reaction) (3 points)
- Polymorphonuclear percentage (PMN%) >80% (2 points)

Major criteria (at least one of the following)				Decision
Two positive cultures of the same organism				Infected
Sinus tract with evidence of communication to the joint or visualization of the prosthesis				
Preoperative Diagnosis		Minor Criteria	Score	Decision
	Serum	Elevated CRP or D-Dimer	2	≥ 6 Infected 2–5 Possibly Infected[a] 0–1 Not Infected
		Elevated ESR	1	
	Synovial	Elevated synovial WBC count or LE	3	
		Positive alpha-defensin	3	
		Elevated synovial PMN (%)	2	
		Elevated synovial CRP	1	
Intraoperative Diagnosis		Inconclusive pre-op score or dry tap[a]	Score	Decision
		Preoperative score	—	≥ 6 Infected 4–5 Inconclusive[b] ≤3 Not Infected
		Positive histology	3	
		Positive purulence	3	
		Single positive culture	2	

[a]For patients with inconclusive minor criteria, operative criteria can also be used to fulfill the definition of PJI.
[b]Consider further molecular diagnostics such as next-generation sequencing.
CRP, C-reactive protein; ESR, erythrocyte sedimentation rate; LE, leukocyte esterase; PMN, polymorphonuclear; WBC, white blood cell.

Table 1.
New scoring-based definition for periprosthetic joint infection (PJI). Proceed with caution in: adverse local tissue reactions, crystal deposition disease, and slow-growing organisms.

- Synovial CRP >6.9 mg/L (1 point)
- Intraoperative findings:
- Positive histological analysis (3 points)
- Presence of purulence (3 points)
- Single positive culture (2 points)

Patients achieving a combined score of ≥6 are classified as infected, while scores between 2 and 5 require intraoperative findings for a definitive diagnosis. Scores ≤3 are indicative of no infection. This scoring system represents a significant advancement in standardizing PJI diagnosis, though further validation and refinement are ongoing to enhance clinical applicability (**Table 1**).

5. Clinical diagnosis

The clinical diagnosis of PJI presents considerable challenges, as the clinical manifestations can often be subtle, particularly in chronic cases. Furthermore, other mechanisms of arthroplasty failure may coexist with PJI, complicating the diagnostic process [21]. Acute PJI, however, typically exhibits more distinct clinical features, including joint pain, erythema, localized warmth, cellulitis, wound discharge, and fever. These signs are more pronounced during acute infections compared to chronic presentations.

Pain remains the most common presenting symptom in PJI, particularly when it occurs at rest or during nighttime. Such presentations should raise a high index of suspicion for infection. Additionally, a history of prolonged wound drainage following surgery in a patient who experiences persistent pain can serve as a critical indicator in establishing the diagnosis [22]. Surgeons must carefully evaluate these clinical signs and symptoms, as they provide valuable context for identifying potential PJI.

6. Laboratory diagnosis

Laboratory investigations have historically played a crucial role in the diagnosis of PJI. Commonly utilized tests include a complete blood count with differential, ESR, and CRP levels. An ESR exceeding 30 mm/h or a serum CRP level greater than 10 mg/L is suggestive of infection [20]. However, these tests are not definitive; studies have demonstrated a false-positive rate of approximately 15%, particularly in cases involving low-virulence pathogens [23, 24].

Recent research has highlighted the utility of additional laboratory parameters, such as the neutrophil-to-lymphocyte ratio (NLR) and the monocyte-to-lymphocyte ratio (MLR). These ratios are derived from routine complete blood counts and offer a low-cost, readily accessible adjunct for detecting acute PJI. With reasonable diagnostic accuracy, NLR and MLR provide supplementary information to traditional markers, making them valuable tools in the diagnostic workflow [25].

In summary, while laboratory markers such as ESR and CRP remain staples in the diagnostic arsenal, emerging evidence suggests that leveraging additional parameters like NLR and MLR can enhance the accuracy of diagnosing acute PJIs. Integration of these novel approaches into routine practice holds promise for improving diagnostic outcomes.

7. Aspiration and microbiological studies

When clinical signs, symptoms, or serological tests raise suspicion of a PJI, the next step in the diagnostic process often involves joint aspiration. Synovial fluid analysis, particularly when paired with culture studies, plays a vital role in diagnosing PJIs and generally provides more reliable insights than blood tests.

Traditionally, the culture of periprosthetic tissue has been considered the gold standard for diagnosing PJI. Synovial fluid, a sterile biological sample, is highly valuable for microbiological analysis, as any microorganism isolated from this fluid, provided contamination is ruled out, can be deemed a potential pathogen. However, the method's sensitivity is notably low, particularly for detecting low-virulence microorganisms. To enhance sensitivity, the practice of inoculating synovial fluid into blood culture bottles has been adopted, although this technique also struggles to differentiate contamination from genuine infections. To mitigate this issue, guidelines recommend obtaining multiple samples—typically three to six—for separate processing and analysis. According to criteria established by Atkins et al. [26], isolating the same organism in at least three culture samples achieves a specificity of 99.6%. However, culture results can take days to develop and may be affected by factors such as low bacterial load, biofilm presence, prior antibiotic exposure, or contamination [27, 28].

Recent advancements have focused on using synovial biomarkers as supplementary tools to improve diagnostic accuracy [29]. Markers like synovial WBC count, PMN%, and AD are key components of the 2018 International Consensus Meeting (ICM) criteria for diagnosing PJI in hips and knees [30, 31]. Nevertheless, these markers are not without limitations. Synovial WBC and PMN% levels, for example, are susceptible to variability influenced by individual patient factors, coexisting inflammatory conditions [32], or even the presence of prosthetic implants [33]. Optimal thresholds for detecting PJI vary widely, ranging from 1100 to 4200 cells/μL for chronic infections, depending on the joint, microorganism, and laboratory protocols [34–36]. Synovial WBC counts can also yield false-positive results in cases involving inflammatory arthritis or metallosis [37].

Alpha-defensin, a peptide involved in the immune response [38] has emerged as a promising biomarker due to its high sensitivity and specificity in detecting PJI [39, 40]. However, its widespread use is limited by cost—ranging between $500 and $1000 per test—and availability, as not all institutions have access to this diagnostic tool [41, 42]. As such, there is a clear need for biomarkers that are easily accessible, relatively noninvasive, and affordable to improve the accuracy of diagnoses. Similarly, other biomarkers such as synovial leukocyte esterase [36], synovial CRP [43], D-dimer [44], interleukin-6 (IL-6) [45], calprotectin [46], and adenosine [34] have been explored for their diagnostic potential. While many show promise challenges such as cost, specialized equipment requirements, and institutional accessibility limit their routine clinical use [47].

In cases where synovial fluid cannot be aspirated—a scenario known as a "dry tap"—the absence of fluid does not rule out infection [48]. Studies have demonstrated that saline lavage of the joint capsule, followed by culture of the recovered fluid, can provide valuable diagnostic information. For instance, one investigation reported that saline lavage cultures achieved 83% sensitivity, 93% specificity, and 83% overall accuracy compared with tissue cultures obtained during revision surgery. This technique offers an alternative diagnostic pathway when standard aspiration methods are unsuccessful [49].

Recent studies have also identified synovial absolute neutrophil count (ANC) as a valuable diagnostic parameter, particularly for acute PJI [50, 51]. For example, specific ANC thresholds for hip and knee PJIs have been established, with higher values typically observed in acute infections due to a stronger immune response compared to chronic infections [16]. Research has demonstrated optimal ANC cut-offs of 3249 cells/μL for hip PJIs within 6 weeks postoperatively and 25,645 cells/μL for cases occurring 6–12 weeks postoperatively [51]. For knee PJIs, thresholds of 8346 and 1684 cells/μL have been identified for the same respective timeframes, with corresponding sensitivities and specificities exceeding 80% [50]. These variances in the optimal thresholds are intuitive, as an acute PJI generally triggers a more robust immune response than a chronic infection.

While biomarkers such as alpha-defensin and novel synovial markers show promise, their high costs and limited accessibility underscore the need for affordable, widely available diagnostic tools. Future research into accessible biomarkers and optimized diagnostic protocols will be pivotal in enhancing the accuracy and efficiency of PJI diagnosis.

8. Radiographic evaluation

Radiographic assessment can provide valuable insights when evaluating a suspected PJI. Specific findings, such as radiolucent lines, focal osteolysis, and periosteal bone formation, may support the diagnosis. Among these, periosteal bone formation is particularly indicative of a deep periprosthetic infection, given its strong correlation with this condition. However, other radiographic signs, such as radiolucent lines, often fail to distinguish between aseptic and septic loosening, limiting their diagnostic utility. Similarly, endosteal erosions around the femoral canal, while commonly observed, can occur in both aseptic and septic loosening, further complicating interpretation.

The absence of radiographic abnormalities does not exclude the possibility of infection, underscoring the need for a comprehensive diagnostic approach. Advanced imaging modalities, such as nuclear scintigraphy, are occasionally employed, though their role in confirming PJI remains less clearly defined. Nuclear scintigraphy, using either technetium-99 m or gallium-67-labeled white blood cell scans, demonstrates high sensitivity but low specificity in detecting PJIs [52]. These scans identify inflammation within periprosthetic tissues, but this characteristic also makes them prone to false positives. For example, inflammation caused by periprosthetic bone remodeling within 12 months postoperatively or aseptic loosening due to prosthesis movement can mimic the findings of infection.

While radiographic evaluation contributes to the diagnostic process, its limitations necessitate the integration of radiologic findings with clinical, laboratory, and microbiological data to achieve an accurate diagnosis of PJI.

9. Intraoperative diagnosis of PJI

The presence of gross purulence observed during surgery can provide strong evidence of a PJI. However, in many cases, even experienced surgeons may find it challenging to make a definitive intraoperative diagnosis based solely on gross findings. This underscores the importance of utilizing additional diagnostic tools during revision arthroplasty.

Histopathological examination of periprosthetic tissue samples is a highly reliable method for diagnosing PJI when performed by a pathologist with expertise in interpreting such tissue. Despite its diagnostic value, histological analysis of intra-articular samples, such as frozen sections, is not universally available and may not be routinely performed at all institutions [53]. However, when accessible, intraoperative histopathological evaluation should be considered, particularly in cases where infection is suspected based on clinical judgment. The results can significantly influence surgical management decisions, such as determining whether to perform a one-stage or two-stage revision arthroplasty.

To optimize the likelihood of identifying the causative microorganism, it is recommended to collect at least three, and ideally five to six, periprosthetic tissue samples during surgery. These samples, along with the explanted prosthesis, should be submitted for both aerobic and anaerobic cultures. This approach maximizes the diagnostic yield and ensures a comprehensive microbiological evaluation, which is essential for guiding targeted antimicrobial therapy and surgical planning.

10. Management of infection

The choice of the optimal treatment strategy for managing PJIs depends on a range of critical factors. These include the timing of infection onset, the duration of symptoms, the condition of the local soft tissues, the number of prior surgical interventions, and the identification and characteristics of the causative pathogen. The pathogen's virulence, antibiotic susceptibility, and resistance profile play a pivotal role in guiding treatment options. Additionally, patient-specific factors, such as underlying comorbidities, must be carefully considered to tailor the therapeutic approach and improve outcomes.

11. Debridement, implant retention, and antibiotics therapy (DAIR)

Debridement, antibiotics, and implant retention (DAIR) is a primary treatment approach for acute PJI and should be performed promptly following symptom onset. This procedure is relatively straightforward and offers several advantages, including lower morbidity, shorter hospital stays, and reduced costs compared to revision surgery. However, the reported success rates for DAIR, particularly when combined with prolonged antibiotic therapy, vary widely in the literature, ranging from 21 to 89% [54]. More recent studies have reported higher success rates, with eradication rates reaching 92.8% [55, 56].

The variability in outcomes highlights the importance of several factors in determining treatment success. Key contributors to failure include prolonged symptom duration, a longer interval since the initial arthroplasty, the need for repeated debridement procedures, and the characteristics of the infecting microorganism. Specific pathogens, such as *Staphylococcus* species, are associated with higher failure rates, particularly when combined with limited antibiotic options or resistance. Additional risk factors include a high American Society of Anesthesiologists (ASA) score and intra-articular purulence [57]. Furthermore, patient-related factors, such as comorbidities, soft tissue integrity, and bone stock quality, significantly influence the feasibility of DAIR and its likelihood of success.

DAIR should be reserved for carefully selected patients. When specific conditions are met, its success rates are comparable to those of exchange arthroplasty. The criteria for optimal DAIR outcomes include (1) a stable implant, (2) the presence of a pathogen that is susceptible to antibiotics effective against biofilm-forming microorganisms, and (3) an infection duration of fewer than 4–6 weeks. Patients with early-onset infections or late acute-onset hematogenous infections often qualify for this procedure [55, 56]. Selecting adequate antibiotics and their optimal period for treating PJIs remains a challenge, yet these factors are crucial in accomplishing prosperous debridement consequences. Culture findings are frequently used to guide the selection of antibiotics; for staphylococcal infections, rifampicin is frequently advised. However, there is not enough solid evidence to support antibiotic selection when culture data are unavailable.

The choice and duration of antibiotic therapy are critical determinants of DAIR outcomes, although optimal regimens remain uncertain. Antibiotic selection is typically guided by culture results, with rifampin often used in combination therapy for *Staphylococcus* infections due to its efficacy against biofilm-associated bacteria. However, there is limited evidence regarding the ideal antibiotics for cases where cultures are not yet available. Vancomycin is frequently considered a viable option, though definitive recommendations for empirical therapy cannot be made at this time.

The duration of antibiotic treatment varies widely, from 6 weeks to 6 months, and adjustments should be based on microbiological findings and clinical response.

Subtherapeutic antibiotic levels may allow residual bacteria to survive and eventually re-establish a biofilm, serving as a persistent nidus for infection. Controlled-release antibiotic delivery systems, while capable of achieving high local concentrations, often exhibit a rapid decline in drug levels below the minimum inhibitory concentration (MIC), raising concerns about the emergence of resistant strains. Conversely, excessively high antibiotic concentrations may interfere with stem cell recruitment, osteoblast activity, and osteointegration, potentially impairing prosthesis stability and bone healing.

In summary, DAIR is a viable treatment option for well-selected patients with acute PJI, provided that surgical and antibiotic strategies are carefully tailored to the individual case. Continued research into optimal antibiotic regimens and delivery methods is essential for improving long-term outcomes.

12. One-stage revision

One-stage revision, also known as direct exchange arthroplasty, offers significant advantages in managing infections following total joint arthroplasty (TJA). This approach involves a single surgical procedure in which the infected prosthesis is removed, the joint is thoroughly debrided, and a new implant is placed during the same operation. By completing the revision in one procedure, patients face reduced cumulative perioperative risks compared to two-stage revision. Additionally, the absence of temporary spacers eliminates the complications associated with their use, leading to fewer overall surgical challenges.

From a financial and resource allocation perspective, one-stage revision is inherently more cost-effective than a two-stage procedure when successful. However, the cost-benefit ratio becomes less clear when factoring in the potential for increased failure rates associated with this approach. Determining the economic impact of one-stage revisions requires balancing the lower upfront costs against the potential need for additional interventions in cases of failure.

A review of the literature highlights several factors linked to the success of one-stage revisions:

1. The absence of wound complications following the initial TJA.

2. The patient's overall good health.

3. The presence of antibiotic-sensitive pathogens, particularly Staphylococcus or Streptococcus species.

4. The use of antibiotics incorporated into cement that effectively targets the identified organisms.

Additionally, Citak et al. [58] revealed that certain factors are associated with higher failure rates following one-stage revision, including (**Table 2**):

1. Weight $\geq$ 100 kg

2. History of Deep vein thrombosis, >4 operations, Polymicrobial infection, One-stage exchange due to periprosthetic joint infection, Two-stage exchange due to periprosthetic joint infection

Risk Factor
• Weight ≥100 kg
• History;
• Deep vein thrombosis
• >4 operations
• Polymicrobial infection
• One-stage exchange due to periprosthetic joint infection
• Two-stage exchange due to periprosthetic joint infection
• Surgery time > 4 hours
• Persistent wound drainage
• Wound revision due to healing disorders
• Isolation of Streptococcus
• Isolation of Enterococcus

Table 2.
The risk factors associated with higher failure rate following one-stage septic revision arthroplasty.

3. Surgery time > 4 hours

4. Persistent wound drainage

5. Wound revision due to healing disorders

6. Isolation of Streptococcus

7. Isolation of Enterococcus

One-stage revision can be an effective treatment option for carefully selected patients, particularly when the infecting organisms are sensitive to available antibiotics and the patient's overall health supports recovery. Further research is needed to refine patient selection criteria and optimize protocols for this approach.

13. Two-stage revision

Two-stage revision is widely regarded as the gold standard for managing PJIs, particularly in TJA. This approach is designed to ensure complete eradication of the infection while achieving consistently high success rates. The procedure involves two distinct stages: the initial debridement and removal of the infected implant, followed by the placement of an antibiotic-loaded spacer. The second stage involves reimplantation of a new prosthesis after infection control is confirmed.

The advantages of two-stage revision are numerous. The removal of infected components and aggressive debridement expose any residual bacteria embedded in the biofilm, allowing for their eradication. Antibiotic-eluting spacers provide localized delivery of high concentrations of antibiotics, enhancing the treatment's efficacy. Articulating spacers offer additional benefits, including partial joint mobility, preservation of limb length, and maintenance of soft tissue tension between stages, ultimately improving functional outcomes. Despite these advantages, several questions remain regarding the timing of antibiotic administration, the optimal use of articulating spacers, and the appropriate interval before reimplantation.

Two-stage revision is generally regarded as the gold standard for the treatment of infected THA. Two-stage revisions boast eradication rates exceeding 90%, underscoring their reliability [59]. The fundamental principles of this procedure involve the complete removal of all prosthetic components and cement, combined with radical debridement of infected tissues and bone. However, challenges persist, particularly in treating resistant microorganisms. Antibiotic resistance is an emerging concern, as more patients present with complex, difficult-to-eradicate infections. For instance, Salgado et al. reported a 50% failure rate among 12 patients with MRSA infections [60]. Similarly, Kilgus et al. documented a 48% success rate in 19 cases of resistant bacterial infections where antibiotic-loaded cement was not utilized during two-stage reimplantation [61]. Uchiyama et al. observed reinfection in 10 of 31 hips (32.3%) following staged reimplantation with antibiotic-impregnated cement spacers [62]. Although studies have demonstrated that antibiotic levels within spacers can remain above the MIC for common pathogens for several months postimplantation, the hydrophobic nature of bone cement limits effective antibiotic elution to approximately 10% of its total content [59, 63]. This limitation underscores the need for further advancements in spacer technology and antibiotic delivery methods to improve outcomes, particularly in cases involving resistant pathogens.

While two-stage revision remains a highly effective strategy for treating PJIs, its success can be influenced by factors such as the resistance profile of the infecting bacteria, the use of antibiotic-loaded spacers, and the timing of reimplantation. Continued research and refinement of this approach are essential to address these challenges and enhance treatment outcomes.

14. Conclusion

Diagnosing PJI necessitates a structured and systematic approach. The diagnostic process typically begins with sensitive blood tests, such as CRP and ESR, which help to exclude or suggest the presence of PJI. This is followed by joint fluid aspiration to confirm the diagnosis, as outlined by the current American Academy of Orthopedic Surgeons (AAOS) guidelines. Synovial fluid analysis, including cell count, differential, and culture, remains a cornerstone of diagnostic accuracy in this context.

Despite the availability of standardized diagnostic criteria and numerous testing modalities, a unified consensus on the optimal diagnostic approach remains elusive. Established frameworks, such as those proposed by the MSIS and subsequent updates, have advanced the field by offering evidence-based protocols. However, their application in daily clinical practice is often met with variability, reflecting ongoing debates and gaps in standardization.

The management of PJI remains one of the most complex and challenging complications associated with total joint arthroplasty. Despite significant advancements in evidence-based strategies, treatment outcomes are still limited by issues such as antibiotic resistance, biofilm-associated infections, and the intricacies of surgical decision-making. The lack of universally agreed-upon standard procedures in the literature further complicates clinical practice.

Given these challenges, adopting a multidisciplinary approach is essential for the effective management of patients with PJI. Collaboration among orthopedic surgeons, infectious disease specialists, microbiologists, pathologists, and radiologists is critical to optimizing diagnosis and treatment. This team-based approach ensures that all facets of the patient's condition—including infection control, surgical management, and long-term functional outcomes—are addressed comprehensively.

Author details

Taner Karlidag* and Omer Halit Keskin
Department of Orthopedics and Traumatology, Gaziantep City Hospital, Gaziantep, Turkey

*Address all correspondence to: dr.tanerkarlidag@gmail.com

References

[1] Shahi A, Tan TL, Chen AF, Maltenfort MG, Parvizi J. In-hospital mortality in patients with periprosthetic joint infection. The Journal of Arthroplasty. 2017;**32**:948-952.e1. DOI: 10.1016/j.arth.2016.09.027

[2] Boddapati V, Fu MC, Tetreault MW, Blevins JL, Richardson SS, Su EP. Short-term complications after revision hip arthroplasty for prosthetic joint infection are increased relative to noninfectious revisions. The Journal of Arthroplasty. 2018;**33**:2997-3002. DOI: 10.1016/j.arth.2018.05.001

[3] Helwig P, Morlock J, Oberst M, Hauschild O, Hübner J, Borde J, et al. Periprosthetic joint infection—Effect on quality of life. International Orthopaedics. 2014;**38**:1077-1081. DOI: 10.1007/s00264-013-2265-y

[4] Ramalhete R, Brown R, Blunn G, Skinner J, Coathup M, Graney I, et al. A novel antimicrobial coating to prevent periprosthetic joint infection. Bone and Joint Research. 2020;**9**:848-856. DOI: 10.1302/2046-3758.912.BJR-2020-0157.R1

[5] Ahmed SS, Haddad FS. Prosthetic joint infection. Bone and Joint Research. 2019;**8**:570-572. DOI: 10.1302/2046-3758.812.BJR-2019-0340

[6] Bozic KJ, Kurtz SM, Lau E, Ong K, Chiu V, Vail TP, et al. The epidemiology of revision total knee arthroplasty in the United States. Clinical Orthopaedics and Related Research. 2010;**468**:45-51. DOI: 10.1007/s11999-009-0945-0

[7] Bozic KJ, Kurtz SM, Lau E, Ong K, Vail TP, Berry DJ. The epidemiology of revision total hip arthroplasty in the United States. The Journal of Bone and Joint Surgery-American. 2009;**91**:128-133. DOI: 10.2106/JBJS.H.00155

[8] Premkumar A, Kolin DA, Farley KX, Wilson JM, McLawhorn AS, Cross MB, et al. Projected economic burden of periprosthetic joint infection of the hip and knee in the United States. The Journal of Arthroplasty. 2021;**36**:1484-1489.e3. DOI: 10.1016/j.arth.2020.12.005

[9] Schwartz AM, Farley KX, Guild GN, Bradbury TL. Projections and epidemiology of revision hip and knee arthroplasty in the United States to 2030. The Journal of Arthroplasty. 2020;**35**:S79-S85. DOI: 10.1016/j.arth.2020.02.030

[10] Xu C, Tan TL, Kuo F-C, Goswami K, Wang Q, Parvizi J. Reevaluating current cutoffs for acute periprosthetic joint infection: Current thresholds are insensitive. The Journal of Arthroplasty. 2019;**34**:2744-2748. DOI: 10.1016/j.arth.2019.06.048

[11] Goswami K, Parvizi J, Maxwell CP. Current recommendations for the diagnosis of acute and chronic PJI for hip and knee—Cell counts, alpha-Defensin, leukocyte esterase, next-generation sequencing. Current Reviews in Musculoskeletal Medicine. 2018;**11**:428-438. DOI: 10.1007/s12178-018-9513-0

[12] Tsukayama DT, Estrada R, Gustilo RB. Infection after total hip arthroplasty. A study of the treatment of one hundred and six infections*. Journal of Bone and Joint Surgery. 1996;**78**:512-523. DOI: 10.2106/00004623-199604000-00005

[13] Senthi S, Munro JT, Pitto RP. Infection in total hip replacement: Meta-analysis. International Orthopaedics.

2011;**35**:253-260. DOI: 10.1007/s00264-010-1144-z

[14] Parvizi J, Ghanem E, Sharkey P, Aggarwal A, Burnett SRJ, Barrack RL. Diagnosis of infected total knee: Findings of a multicenter database. Clinical Orthopaedics and Related Research. 2008;**466**:2628-2633. DOI: 10.1007/s11999-008-0471-5

[15] Akkaya M, Zanna L, Sangaletti R, Bokhari A, Gehrke T, Citak M. What is the most reliable concordance rate of preoperative synovial fluid aspiration and intraoperative biopsy to detect periprosthetic joint infection in knee, hip and shoulder Arthroplasty? Antibiotics. 2023;**12**:1482. DOI: 10.3390/antibiotics12101482

[16] Karlidag T, Luo TD, Gehrke T, Citak M. How reliable is the absolute synovial polymorphonuclear neutrophil cell count in diagnosing periprosthetic joint infection? The Journal of Arthroplasty. 2024;**39**:1060-1068. DOI: 10.1016/j.arth.2023.10.038

[17] Osmon DR, Berbari EF, Berendt AR, Lew D, Zimmerli W, Steckelberg JM, et al. Executive summary: Diagnosis and management of prosthetic joint infection: Clinical practice guidelines by the infectious diseases Society of America. Clinical Infectious Diseases. 2013;**56**:1-10. DOI: 10.1093/cid/cis966

[18] Parvizi J, Zmistowski B, Berbari EF, Bauer TW, Springer BD, Della Valle CJ, et al. New definition for periprosthetic joint infection: From the workgroup of the musculoskeletal infection society. Clinical Orthopaedics and Related Research. 2011;**469**:2992-2994. DOI: 10.1007/s11999-011-2102-9

[19] Parvizi J, Gehrke T, Chen AF. Proceedings of the international consensus on periprosthetic joint infection. The Bone and Joint Journal. 2013;**95-B**:1450-1452. DOI: 10.1302/0301-620X.95B11.33135

[20] Parvizi J, Tan TL, Goswami K, Higuera C, Della Valle C, Chen AF, et al. The 2018 definition of periprosthetic hip and knee infection: An evidence-based and validated criteria. The Journal of Arthroplasty. 2018;**33**:1309-1314.e2. DOI: 10.1016/j.arth.2018.02.078

[21] Karlidag T, Zanna L, Traverso G, Lee M-J, Gehrke T, Citak M. Assessing the reliability of automated cell count analysis of synovial fluid in the setting of revision total knee arthroplasty. Archives of Orthopaedic and Trauma Surgery. 2024;**145**:25. DOI: 10.1007/s00402-024-05652-4

[22] Abdelaziz H, Grüber H, Gehrke T, Salber J, Citak M. What are the factors associated with re-revision after one-stage revision for periprosthetic joint infection of the hip? A case-control study. Clinical Orthopaedics and Related Research. 2019;**477**:2258-2263. DOI: 10.1097/CORR.0000000000000780

[23] Akgün D, Müller M, Perka C, Winkler T. The serum level of C-reactive protein alone cannot be used for the diagnosis of prosthetic joint infections, especially in those caused by organisms of low virulence. The Bone and Joint Journal. 2018;**100-B**:1482-1486. DOI: 10.1302/0301-620X.100B11.BJJ-2018-0514.R1

[24] Kheir MM, Tan TL, Shohat N, Foltz C, Parvizi J. Routine diagnostic tests for periprosthetic joint infection demonstrate a high false-negative rate and are influenced by the infecting organism. Journal of Bone and Joint Surgery. 2018;**100**:2057-2065. DOI: 10.2106/JBJS.17.01429

[25] Karlidag T, Dasci MF, Steinhoff J, Gehrke T, Citak M. What is the diagnostic accuracy of neutrophil to lymphocyte ratio and monocyte to lymphocyte ratio in detecting acute periprosthetic joint infections? A gender-specific analysis. Archives of Orthopaedic and Trauma Surgery. 2023;**144**:5071-5078. DOI: 10.1007/s00402-023-05162-9

[26] Atkins BL, Athanasou N, Deeks JJ, Crook DWM, Simpson H, Peto TEA, et al. Prospective evaluation of criteria for microbiological diagnosis of prosthetic-joint infection at revision arthroplasty. Journal of Clinical Microbiology. 1998;**36**:2932-2939. DOI: 10.1128/JCM.36.10.2932-2939.1998

[27] Cai Y, Liang J, Chen X, Zhang G, Jing Z, Zhang R, et al. Synovial fluid neutrophil extracellular traps could improve the diagnosis of periprosthetic joint infection. Bone and Joint Research. 2023;**12**:113-120. DOI: 10.1302/2046-3758.122.BJR-2022-0391.R1

[28] Zanna L, Sangaletti R, Akkaya M, Shen T, Abuljadail S, Gehrke T, et al. What is the concordance rate of preoperative synovial fluid aspiration and intraoperative biopsy in detecting periprosthetic joint infection of the shoulder? Journal of Shoulder and Elbow Surgery. 2023;**32**:492-499. DOI: 10.1016/j.jse.2022.10.008

[29] Seetharam A, Dilley JE, Meneghini RM, Kheir MM. Diagnostic utility and thresholds for commonly obtained serum and synovial markers prior to reimplantation in periprosthetic joint infection. The Journal of Arthroplasty. 2023;**38**:1356-1362. DOI: 10.1016/j.arth.2023.01.021

[30] Parvizi J, Gehrke T. Definition of periprosthetic joint infection. The Journal of Arthroplasty. 2014;**29**:1331. DOI: 10.1016/j.arth.2014.03.009

[31] Shohat N, Bauer T, Buttaro M, Budhiparama N, Cashman J, Della Valle CJ, et al. Hip and knee section, what is the definition of a periprosthetic joint infection (PJI) of the knee and the hip? Can the same criteria be used for both joints?: Proceedings of international consensus on orthopedic infections. The Journal of Arthroplasty. 2019;**34**:S325-S327. DOI: 10.1016/j.arth.2018.09.045

[32] Fuchs M, Kirchhoff F, Reichel H, Perka C, Faschingbauer M, Gwinner C. Variation of synovial fluid leucocyte cell count and polymorphonuclear percentage in patients with aseptic revision total knee arthroplasty. Bone and Joint Open. 2021;**2**:576-582. DOI: 10.1302/2633-1462.28.BJO-2021-0109

[33] Deirmengian CA, Kazarian GS, Feeley SP, Sizer SC. False-positive automated synovial fluid white blood cell counting is a concern for both hip and knee arthroplasty aspirates. The Journal of Arthroplasty. 2020;**35**:S304-S307. DOI: 10.1016/j.arth.2020.01.060

[34] Sousa R, Serrano P, Gomes Dias J, Oliveira JC, Oliveira A. Improving the accuracy of synovial fluid analysis in the diagnosis of prosthetic joint infection with simple and inexpensive biomarkers. Bone and Joint Journal. 2017;**99-B**:351-7. DOI: 10.1302/0301-620X.99B3.BJJ-2016-0684.R1

[35] Ottink KD, Strahm C, Muller-Kobold A, Sendi P, Wouthuyzen-Bakker M. Factors to consider when assessing the diagnostic accuracy of synovial leukocyte count in periprosthetic joint infection. Journal of Bone and Joint Infection. 2019;**4**:167-173. DOI: 10.7150/jbji.34854

[36] Zahar A, Lausmann C, Cavalheiro C, Dhamangaonkar AC, Bonanzinga T,

Gehrke T, et al. How reliable is the cell count analysis in the diagnosis of prosthetic joint infection? The Journal of Arthroplasty. 2018;**33**:3257-3262. DOI: 10.1016/j.arth.2018.05.018

[37] Qin L, Wang H, Zhao C, Chen C, Chen H, Li X, et al. Serum and synovial biomarkers for distinguishing between chronic periprosthetic joint infections and rheumatoid arthritis: A prospective cohort study. The Journal of Arthroplasty. 2022;**37**:342-346. DOI: 10.1016/j.arth.2021.09.009

[38] Sigmund IK, Holinka J, Gamper J, Staats K, Böhler C, Kubista B, et al. Qualitative α-defensin test (Synovasure) for the diagnosis of periprosthetic infection in revision total joint arthroplasty. Bone and Joint Journal. 2017;**99-B**:66-72. DOI: 10.1302/0301-620X.99B1.BJJ-2016-0295.R1

[39] Deirmengian C, Kardos K, Kilmartin P, Cameron A, Schiller K, Booth RE, et al. The alpha-defensin test for periprosthetic joint infection outperforms the leukocyte esterase test strip. Clinical Orthopaedics and Related Research. 2015;**473**:198-203. DOI: 10.1007/s11999-014-3722-7

[40] Bingham J, Clarke H, Spangehl M, Schwartz A, Beauchamp C, Goldberg B. The alpha defensin-1 biomarker assay can be used to evaluate the potentially infected total joint arthroplasty. Clinical Orthopaedics and Related Research. 2014;**472**:4006-4009. DOI: 10.1007/s11999-014-3900-7

[41] Kleiss S, Jandl NM, Novo de Oliveira A, Rüther W, Niemeier A. Diagnostic accuracy of alpha-defensin enzyme-linked immunosorbent assay in the clinical evaluation of painful hip and knee arthroplasty with possible prosthetic joint infection. Bone and Joint Journal. 2019;**101-B**:970-977. DOI: 10.1302/0301-620X.101B8.BJJ-2018-1390.R2

[42] Kleeman-Forsthuber LT, Johnson RM, Brady AC, Pollet AK, Dennis DA, Jennings JM. Alpha-defensin offers limited utility in routine workup of periprosthetic joint infection. The Journal of Arthroplasty. 2021;**36**:1746-1752. DOI: 10.1016/j.arth.2020.12.018

[43] Buttaro MA, Martorell G, Quinteros M, Comba F, Zanotti G, Piccaluga F. Intraoperative synovial C-reactive protein is as useful as frozen section to detect periprosthetic hip infection. Clinical Orthopaedics and Related Research. 2015;**473**:3876-3881. DOI: 10.1007/s11999-015-4340-8

[44] Shahi A, Kheir MM, Tarabichi M, Hosseinzadeh HRS, Tan TL, Parvizi J. Serum D-dimer test is promising for the diagnosis of periprosthetic joint infection and timing of reimplantation. Journal of Bone and Joint Surgery. 2017;**99**:1419-1427. DOI: 10.2106/JBJS.16.01395

[45] Lenski M, Scherer MA. Synovial IL-6 AS inflammatory marker in periprosthetic joint infections. The Journal of Arthroplasty. 2014;**29**:1105-1109. DOI: 10.1016/j.arth.2014.01.014

[46] Wouthuyzen-Bakker M, Ploegmakers JJW, Ottink K, Kampinga GA, Wagenmakers-Huizenga L, Jutte PC, et al. Synovial calprotectin: An inexpensive biomarker to exclude a chronic prosthetic joint infection. The Journal of Arthroplasty. 2018;**33**:1149-1153. DOI: 10.1016/j.arth.2017.11.006

[47] Tirumala V, Klemt C, Xiong L, Chen W, van den Kieboom J, Kwon Y-M. Diagnostic utility of platelet count/lymphocyte count ratio and platelet count/mean platelet volume ratio in periprosthetic joint infection following

total knee arthroplasty. The Journal of Arthroplasty. 2021;**36**:291-297. DOI: 10.1016/j.arth.2020.07.038

[48] Christensen TH, Ong J, Lin D, Aggarwal VK, Schwarzkopf R, Rozell JC. How does a "dry tap" impact the accuracy of preoperative aspiration results in predicting chronic periprosthetic joint infection? The Journal of Arthroplasty. 2022;**37**:925-929. DOI: 10.1016/j.arth.2022.01.066

[49] Ali F, Wilkinson JM, Cooper JR, Kerry RM, Hamer AJ, Norman P, et al. Accuracy of joint aspiration for the preoperative diagnosis of infection in total hip arthroplasty. The Journal of Arthroplasty. 2006;**21**:221-226. DOI: 10.1016/j.arth.2005.05.027

[50] Uvodich ME, Dugdale EM, Osmon DR, Pagnano MW, Berry DJ, Abdel MP. The effectiveness of laboratory tests to predict early postoperative periprosthetic infection after total knee arthroplasty. Bone and Joint Journal. 2021;**103-B**:177-84. DOI: 10.1302/0301-620X.103B6.BJJ-2020-2397.R1

[51] Dugdale EM, Uvodich ME, Osmon DR, Pagnano MW, Berry DJ, Abdel MP. Laboratory value effectiveness in predicting early postoperative periprosthetic joint infection after total hip arthroplasty. The Journal of Arthroplasty. 2022;**37**:574-580. DOI: 10.1016/j.arth.2021.11.007

[52] Smith SL, Wastie ML, Forster I. Radionuclide bone scintigraphy in the detection of significant complications after total knee joint replacement. Clinical Radiology. 2001;**56**:221-224. DOI: 10.1053/crad.2000.0620

[53] Della VC, Parvizi J, Bauer TW, DiCesare PE, Evans RP, Segreti J, et al. Diagnosis of periprosthetic joint infections of the hip and knee. American Academy of Orthopaedic The Surgeon. 2010;**18**:760-770. DOI: 10.5435/00124635-201012000-00006

[54] Di Benedetto P, Di Benedetto ED, Salviato D, Beltrame A, Gissoni R, Cainero V, et al. Acute periprosthetic knee infection: Is there still a role for DAIR? Acta Biomed. 2017;**88**:84-91. DOI: 10.23750/abm.v88i2-S.6518

[55] Longo UG, De Salvatore S, Bandini B, Lalli A, Barillà B, Budhiparama NC, et al. Debridement, antibiotics, and implant retention (DAIR) for the early prosthetic joint infection of total knee and hip arthroplasties: A systematic review. Journal of ISAKOS. 2024;**9**:62-70. DOI: 10.1016/j.jisako.2023.09.003

[56] Salman LA, Altahtamouni SB, Khatkar H, Al-Ani A, Ahmed G. Success rate of single versus multiple debridement, antibiotics, and implant retention (DAIR) in hip and knee periprosthetic joint infection: A systematic review and meta-analysis. European Journal of Orthopaedic Surgery and Traumatology. 2024;**34**:3859-3872. DOI: 10.1007/s00590-024-04091-6

[57] Kong L, Cao J, Zhang Y, Ding W, Shen Y. Risk factors for periprosthetic joint infection following primary total hip or knee arthroplasty: A meta-analysis. International Wound Journal. 2017;**14**:529-536. DOI: 10.1111/iwj.12640

[58] Citak M, Friedenstab J, Abdelaziz H, Suero EM, Zahar A, Salber J, et al. Risk factors for failure after 1-stage exchange total knee arthroplasty in the management of periprosthetic joint infection. Journal of Bone and Joint Surgery. 2019;**101**:1061-1069. DOI: 10.2106/JBJS.18.00947

[59] Masri BA, Panagiotopoulos KP, Greidanus NV, Garbuz DS, Duncan CP.

Cementless two-stage exchange arthroplasty for infection after total hip arthroplasty. The Journal of Arthroplasty. 2007;**22**:72-78. DOI: 10.1016/j.arth.2006.02.156

[60] Salgado CD, Dash S, Cantey JR, Marculescu CE. Higher risk of failure of methicillin-resistant staphylococcus aureus prosthetic joint infections. Clinical Orthopaedics and Related Research. 2007;**461**:48-53. DOI: 10.1097/BLO.0b013e3181123d4e

[61] Kilgus DJ, Howe DJ, Strang A. Results of periprosthetic hip and knee infections caused by resistant bacteria. Clinical Orthopaedics and Related Research. 2002;**404**:116-124. DOI: 10.1097/00003086-200211000-00021

[62] Uchiyama K, Takahira N, Fukushima K, Moriya M, Yamamoto T, Minegishi Y, et al. Two-stage revision total hip arthroplasty for periprosthetic infections using antibiotic-impregnated cement spacers of various types and materials. The Scientific World Journal. 2013;**2013**:5. DOI: 10.1155/2013/147248

[63] DiCicco M, Duong T, Chu A, Jansen SA. Tobramycin and gentamycin elution analysis between two in situ polymerizable orthopedic composites. Journal of Biomedical Materials Research. Part B, Applied Biomaterials. 2003;**65B**:137-149. DOI: 10.1002/jbm.b.10528